It's Never Too Late
Healing Prebirth and Birth At Any Age

MIA KALEF, DC

Foreword by Jaap van der Wal

Red Alder
Denman Island, Canada

RED
ALDER

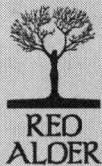

Published by Red Alder
P.O. Box 13
Denman Island, B.C.
VOR 1T0
Canada

Cover image: "Blue Hour Seascape at Galaxidi" by Helen Sotiriadis.
Author photo by Michael Julian Berz
Book and cover design and production by Rayola Creative

The poem "Semen," first appears in *The Taste of Wild Water: Poems and Stories Found While Walking in Woods*, Raven Press, 2009, by permission from the author, Stephen Harrod Buhner.

Red Alder is the first of trees to populate a new or decimated forest. Its roots seed the nourishment for the species yet to come. Works proudly produced through Red Alder serve emerging culture, and ancient or forgotten wisdoms that they stand on.

This book is available in most bookstores, and world-wide through online booksellers.
ISBN: 978-1-7753985-0-9 (print)
ISBN: 978-1-7753985-1-6 (digital)

For all inquiries about this book, please contact the author at mia@miakalef.com

Other title by the author:
The Secret Life of Babies: How Our Prebirth and Birth Experiences Shape Our World

In *It's Never Too Late: Healing Prebirth and Birth At Any Age,* Mia Kalef clearly explains the scientific connections between the intrauterine experience and unexplained physical, mental and emotional symptoms. This seminal work should be required reading for all health professionals, especially those in childbirth and mental health. Whether you need to overcome a difficult birth (as a baby, mother or father), or want to help others prevent, or heal from, them, *It's Never Too Late* is the perfect resource. Reading it will leave you inspired and dedicated to share this profoundly important information with the world.

— Joel M. Evans, M.D., Board Certified OB/GYN
Author, *The Whole Pregnancy Handbook*
Medical Director, Association of Pre and Perinatal Psychology and
Health, Senior Faculty, Institute for Functional Medicine

It's Never Too Late: Healing Prebirth and Birth At Any Age by Mia Kalef is a gentle and profound explanation of early patterns that inform who we are, starting preconception. The text includes science, clinical experience, and healing practices for practitioners, mothers, families, adults and babies. Kalef's voice is expert, kind, and present throughout the book as she addresses the multiple prenatal and perinatal patterns that influence human development. Her consistent message in each chapter is that it is never to late to heal early overwhelming experiences and is a must read for the passionate student in prenatal and perinatal health, or anyone seeking healing and peace.

—Kate White, MA, LMT, RCST®, CEIM, SEP
Director, Center for Prenatal and Perinatal Programs
Director of Education, Association for Prenatal and Perinatal
Psychology and Health

It was around 1974 that I immersed myself for the first time in Pre-, and Peri-Natal Psychology. R. D. Laing, my mentor, was reading Francis J. Mott, who pointed us to Otto Rank, Nandor Fodor, and Stan Grof. Dreams, hypnosis, LSD, Elizabeth Feher's "re-birthing" body-work, Michel Odent's and Frédérick Leboyer's pioneering work — all seemed to point to the importance of early experience in later character formation. To avoid the disbelief and annihilating critique of the establishment, we talked of our discoveries as metaphors, healing stories, helpful myths. In Mia Kalef's book you'll find solid reasons to learn about the actual reality, validity of early learning and patterning for later life. Experience cannot be ignored, even if physics lacks the understanding of the forces which underlie and explain phenomena that influence the quality of our lives. Mia's book is a worthy milestone in this lineage of courageous exploration.

—**Andrew Feldmár, psychologist, psychotherapist**

Our pre-birth and birth experiences create imprints—living memories that have physiological, emotional and spiritual consequences that influence how we relate to the world and to ourselves. Thankfully, if we have challenging early experiences they don't have to define our entire life, if we know what to look for and how to heal these early traumas. Dr. Mia Kalef teaches readers how to discover events that challenged their trust, safety and security within each developmental stage from the point of view of the inner child (starting with conception, then implantation, gestation, birthing and after birth) and how to work with these internalized imprints stuck in the past in now maladaptive contexts so that they can heal.

—**Nancy Eichhorn, PhD,**
Editor of *Somatic Psychotherapy Today*

This is a must read for any one who was born. This book helps us look at deep, old, and habitual patterns that form the core of our being. It is Never Too Late to look at the past to find answers to who we have become based our on pre-conception, conception, pregnancy, birth and early childhood times of development. I was especially intrigued with the chapter that described what happens to mothers and babies who are exposed to common medical birth practices like the use of an epidural, induction and augmentation of labor, the use of forceps and vacuum extractors, and the all-too-common cesarean way of birthing. All of these create an unconscious lasting imprint on the baby and mother that will follow them through life. We do remember birth, and these memories have long term consequences for who we become. Mia does not leave the reader pondering what to do, but offers many beautiful ways to reverse the imprints of these early times of becoming human. I highly recommend *It's Never Too Late* to anyone working with families before stepping into the energy field of another, especially a pregnant, birthing, postpartum mother who is so vulnerable to the energetics around her.

—Barbara Essman, MA,
Director/Owner of The Sacred Birthing School on Kauai

Prenatal Psychology is the most fruitful frontier of human consciousness breached in the last 100 years by Prebirth Pioneers, Explorers and Scientific Researchers.

Dr. Mia Kalef takes her place among of those Pioneers.

The laudatios in the opening pages of Dr. Kalef's book are so accurate we only need say Bravo! Troya & I are filled with appreciation that so many mysteries of exactly how and why we are, as unique personalities, are clearly explained, and with suggested balancing by Dr. Kalef because it is never too late to heal our prebirth and birth imprints."

—Jon RG & Troya GN Turner,
founders of Whole Self Discovery and Development Institute

At last, clinicians and parents have a book of authoritative knowledge that provides a solid foundation for working with the effects of prenatal imprinting. Mia Kalef brings together a clear understanding and set of skills for anyone working in this field and concerned about the lifelong mental and physical health of their smallest and biggest clients. We must all be concerned! Her case studies especially ground the material in the living reality of the treatment room and the heart. This book is an outstanding bridge to help heal all of us with our own early narrative and that of others.

—Michael Shea, PhD,
author of *Biodynamic Craniosacral Therapy Volumes 1 – 5*

To all those yearning to be known

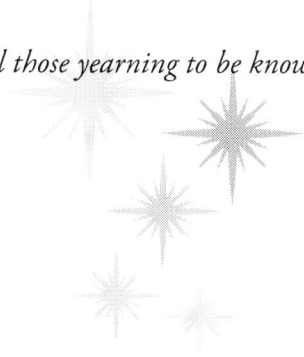

The body came into being through us,
not we from it.
We are as bees, and bodies as honeycomb:
we have made the body,
cell by cell, like wax.

—Rumi

CONTENTS

PART 2: The Imprints

FOREWORD

In the Introduction to this book Mia writes: "I learned the body is an incredible storehouse for events too overwhelming to contend with. I also learned that slowly recovering these memories (in my case largely through craniosacral therapy and other healing modalities) frees us from emotional and physical pain". Memories? Are there memories in a body? Where? And can you treat memories in a body?

I was trained an expert on the prenatal body (embryology) but I still can recall the awkwardness I felt when confronted in the 1980's with psychologists and psychiatrists who referred to prenatal consciousness, using terms like "imprints" and "patterns". These psychotherapists talked about *prenatal experience, fetal psyche, shock of conception* and *somatization.* "Could it be that we pass through transformations or variations of our first prenatal experiences during later cycles of life, even before a special developed nervous system comes in our body? Can it be true that the patterns in our prenatal experiences serve as a kind of template for patterns later forming the tissue of our complex postnatal life of behavior and soul?" (Ronald Laing: *Facts of Life*, 1976).

I had doubts: How could an embryo or fetus possess "mind" or "soul" when it does not even show the simplest features of an actively functioning brain? For most people, the fetus and surely the embryo had become a kind of "half existence", not yet complete yet or at least not entirely "there yet". The embryo was considered to be *mindless,* leading to notions as "not yet *human*" in current moral and ethical debates.

In her current book Mia Kalef searches for how our womb experiences continue to manifest throughout our lives. Are they still there? Where? In the body? How do they feel? How might we recognize them in our children? Can we heal these experiences when they trouble our minds? As a craniosacral therapist, Mia started her quest there where I start also, i.e. in the body. Long ago I started to formulate questions like "What are we actually doing as embryo, when we exist in the womb"? I learned that the shaping of a body is not just past, an embryonic or fetal phase, but it still is our primary and fundamental behavior. The body speaks a (formative) language. Forms are actions, behavior, gestures that can be understood. The widespread scientific paradigm reduces soul, psyche, and personality to brain activity: the worldview of materialism that predominates in science assumes that the body is producing brain activity and that that brain activity is producing our soul, our consciousness, our mind. In this way modern neuropsychologists deny completely that the main domain of our psycho-somatic being and experiencing is the so-called "un-conscious body".

But un-consciousness does not mean "absence of soul or spirit'! "The body developed out of us, not we from it", says Rumi (13th century), "We are bees and our body is a honeycomb. We made the body, cell by cell we made it". This is the kind of truth about the body that I discovered by means of my phenomenological embryology. And if this vision is true, it is easy to imagine that there exist memories, patterns, and imprints held within our bodies from the early life of our bodies. Could we have memories of this prenatal past when we (literally) performed our body (and therefore ourselves)?

Mia Kalef is not following the path which becomes more and more the lazy way of modern psychology — that is, to reduce experiences, feelings, thoughts, consciousness to pure brain processes. That model says for example "Oh, your addiction, your depression, it is simply a biological disorder, it is your hippocampus that does not function well". Instead, Mia, as a truly phenomenological psychotherapist, heals this reductionistic view by "taking for true what your senses are telling you, and how you experience things". This is the method of phenomenology. Of course there is speech of the body; of course shapes and also the functional movements and motions of the body can be understood as gestures, and therefore as behavior and as speech and language. Mia gives the newborn, the infant, and the child, back the language of the body and soul that we are. She invites us not only to observe but also take the other stance and that is: to participate in the nonverbal and (postural) behavior of the child, to give words to that behavior and in this way to listen, to hear and ultimately to understand what a child (or the child in us) might have to tell us about the experiences that she/he had during the so-called unconscious existence in the womb around birth.

I am very impressed how Mia really helps us to communicate with the (wounded) soul of the infant, the not yet verbally equipped child: in order to exchange with each other and to help to find our way back to the experiences, and maybe wounds, that are still there in the unconscious domain of the body and in order to help the child to cope with and find a new balance in the sometimes disturbed equilibrium of the soul. Firmly she persists in the attitude of the phenomenologist: "Although I cannot offer an explanation for the perception babies that young use, I can affirm that I have worked with countless people who report being affected and imprinted by experiences at this early age — even as they are about to be conceived".

The only thing the reader has to do, in order to get contact with the effort of Mia to bring our prenatal consciousness and awareness alive, is to not persist in assuming the habitual role and mind of the traditional scientific onlooker, observer, analyzer. Rather, we are able, as she is doing in this brilliant book, to participate, to share and to tune in with the language and the behavior by which we as adults, as infants, as fetuses, as embryos express our feelings, our hopes, our disappointments, our traumas. Indeed, to help to restore health at any age.

—Jaap van der Wal,
embryologist, phenomenologist, and philosopher
Maastricht, The Netherlands, March 2017

INTRODUCTION

I first began my journey to understanding the roots of physical and emotional challenges twenty years ago, lying on a chiropractic table. At that point I'd suffered with back pain for two years after sustaining an injury while rowing in the national summer games. My crew and I earned a silver medal in that race, but I had to be carried out of the boat, spending the remainder of the season watching from the shore. It was a tough time. Being a teenager unable to continue in the sport I loved left me looking for answers. I spent all the time I would have been training and racing searching for solutions. I went to physiotherapists, a chiropractor, a sports medicine specialist, a rheumatologist, and a traditional bone setter. All of them had interesting perspectives, yet none of them knew what was wrong with me. The explanation I finally was left with was "You have a tissue irritation. We don't know what causes it. It may be with you forever or it may one day leave you."

I gave up looking for answers from the medical world. Within a few months I was able to walk again, but not without tremendous back and leg tension, as well as pounding headaches that would stop me in the middle of a flight of stairs. I was still going to a chiropractor for pain relief, but by this point I was feeling pretty jaded and wasn't expecting much to change. On this day, my chiropractor suggested something new: he would lead me through a guided visualization in the hopes that I might access the reason for my ongoing pain. We had already been through a course of conventional treatment, with some improvement, and he hoped the visualization might take me to a new level.

The visualization was gentle and simple. I was asked to breathe and simply observe what arose in my attention. The further into the visualization I went, the more my body relaxed. For the first time in several years I had no pain. Then I saw myself as a tiny fetus in the womb, and tears involuntarily came to my eyes. At the time I was utterly inexperienced with the world of healing, but what I had just discovered was that emotions were locked away in my body, and by feeling them my body had less pain! A spark was lit that day, one that made me curious about what was at the root of pain, both physical and emotional.

I began to read books about what then was referred to medically as *somatization* — the manifestation of medical conditions with no known physical cause. I came across the works of the late Thomas Hanna and of Wilhelm Reich's protégé Alexander Lowen, and various articles about what then could only be termed mind-body medicine.

My studies and my self-exploration unfolded and eventually revealed trauma from when I was in the womb and during my birth, along with long-buried memories of childhood sexual abuse. I learned the body is an incredible storehouse for events too overwhelming to contend with. I also learned that slowly recovering these memories (in my case largely through craniosacral therapy and other healing modalities) frees us from emotional and physical pain. This journey has continued to intrigue me, and I'm amazed by how much healing is available if we are courageous and curious.

Now, more than twenty five years after that day on the chiropractic table, I work with families and adults who are trying to discover how their early experiences affect them. It still surprises me that in spite of eighty years of scientific data to support the idea that babies are aware as early as conception, and certainly throughout pregnancy, birth, and the first years of life, we still feel it's okay to do things to them and their families as though they're not aware. I find it troubling that we don't treat babies with more respect and care, even though we know unequivocally that they will retain memories of their pre-conception, life in the womb, and their birth, and will develop lasting structural, physiological, emotional, and spiritual consequences from those memories, ranging from low self-esteem and fears to addictions, suicidal behaviours, and other forms of violence.

To put it simply, babies figure that the chemicals, sharp objects, needles, bright lights, loud sounds, and other people's fears and judgments they experience before birth and at birth are cues for what they should expect to experience as they grow. So how can we proceed with the many benefits of our highly developed and useful technological/medical advancements, while protecting the unborn, young babies, and their families from their deleterious effects? If we don't show gentleness, respect for their timing, and an overall reverence for their sovereignty when we use medical interventions, they will replay what we do back to us. The way they love, couple, have children, and, in general, treat other people, will be a replay of how they were thought of and treated before they had words.

In my practice I work with babies and their families, children, and adults to sort out what really happened to them when they were in the womb, being born, and growing as infants. They rediscover the real events that challenged their trust, safety, and security. They also make connections to how these challenges gave rise to their present-day struggles with things like pain, allergies, fears, or habitual isolation. Over and over we discover that these tender and early stages of life are not gone, even though they happened a long time ago. Instead, they persist until the individual can experience the reaction they never got to have. Giving accurate empathy, space for rage and grief, and offering nurturing to those early places allows the person to finally move forward, no matter their age.

The healing work in this book is designed to reunite people of every age with their young, disenfranchised, and still hurting places, and move them forward in the present. Thus, this book is for anyone who wants to explore, discover, and work towards healing the challenges they faced between preconception and just after birth. Although nothing can replace the support of another person or therapist, this book is here to support you in your work at home, on your own, or in between therapeutic sessions. It's also for parents or caregivers who see their child is suffering and are confounded. It's for parents who have been through a challenging birth and are left with the aftereffects of interventions like induction, epidural, forceps, vacuum, cesarean, and separation from their babies. I have also included a small section on healing from miscarriage and other early losses. The profound effects of stillbirth and adoption are not included in this book, as each are worthy of entire books themselves. Fathers and partners are affected by these events, often in equally profound ways, and although I do not use the term "father" or "partner" as often as I do "mother," know that every suggestion in this book (aside from gynecological ones directly related to childbirth) can be used to support fathers or partners as well. Please know that not every baby, child, or adult will exhibit the signs and symptoms I write about in this book. Sometimes they will surprise us and do quite the opposite or something no one would ever expect. My descriptions are possibilities, but not rules, and the tools I offer are to make you a more astute learner of your early self and, if relevant, your child.

My wish for you, the reader, is that you find solace for your struggles, be they with yourself or with your child, or both. Perhaps by reading, your own early sentience will be validated, celebrated, and redeemed. May you find new and non-violent ways to contend with your own or your child's challenges. May whatever coherence you find for yourself also be a gift you can pass along to others you meet on your path. Over time, this type of awareness can spread so babies and their families can do as Nature has offered: experience conception, the time in the womb, birth, and bonding as healthy and whole rites of passage, ones that enliven generations to come. Even though the suffering from challenging pre-birth and birth experiences can be debilitating, Nature has made it so that we all can heal.

Thank you for reading.

PART ONE

Preparing For Our Work

CHAPTER 1

Perspectives

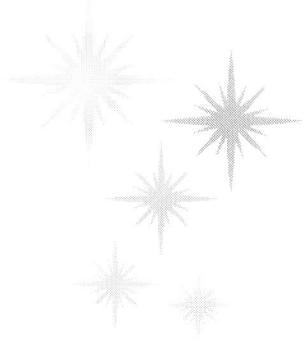

The good news is that healing happens naturally, even without interventions like counselling, bodywork, vitamins, and surgery. But there are circumstances in which the healing process can get bogged down because the challenges are unusually overwhelming. A birth may have so many surprises that we find ourselves rehashing the events for months and even years afterwards. Recurrent pregnancy loss might colour your healthy and sustained pregnancy, making it difficult to celebrate and stay optimistic. Drugs used during pregnancy or birth may confuse your own and your baby's nervous systems, making either or both of you think you should feel flat, nauseous, anxious, or foggy when you try to get together. Years after your own time in the womb, you may still be unsure whether you're wanted due to events back then. These are just a tiny handful of many possible challenges from the pre-birth and birth periods. What gets left over from pre-birth and birth largely heals if we receive consistent, loving attention after birth, and yet some aspects of the challenges will linger. The point of this book is to provide perspectives that will give you greater clarity and help you make connections that will strengthen your or yours and your baby's natural ability to heal. I provide details on what lingers and focus on what ingredients lead to maximal healing from pre-birth and birth, whether it's for you or for you and your baby.

When pain, emotional challenge, disease, or problems at work or in relationships hit, they can feel all-consuming. The conventional places we turn to might have answers, yet often you are left on your own to muddle through whatever is happening. It's normal to have human reactions like fear, anger, and denial. These are standard responses to unusual circumstances. However, even when you have had those initial feelings, it's good to pay attention if feelings are still there. Sometimes you've had your initial response, yet there is more that wants to be explored, felt, and released. Here lies the opportunity in this book.

To give you an example: someone I know, I'll call him Tristan, realized his birth had been very traumatic and was affecting his ability to be close to people. He was separated from his mother in an incubator after birth and had little of the closeness that he needed. He learned to manage by accepting his aloneness, and as he grew older, he would quickly whisk away any desire for closeness as soon as it arose, as though it was not available. You see, for him, it was too painful to be close to someone. He would have to first grieve the horrible feelings of separation he had after his birth. Because babies learn so quickly about the world, this first experience of separation taught him closeness would never be available — even when it was right in front of him in the form of a friend or potential partner. By employing the perspectives in this book and working through some of the exercises, Tristan was better able to make a choice, to determine whether he really wanted to be alone or if he was simply remembering having to be alone even though he wanted closeness. Over years of practice, he was able to grieve the separation from his mother and father, and found he actually wanted to be close to people. Before, he couldn't even see others' offers of closeness because he was so adapted to a world that had no one. After, he noticed gestures of closeness. He no longer believed, or acted like, he was so alone.

You may think Tristan's story is more extreme than what you suspect your baby is dealing with, but it may be too early to tell. Even though babies don't have words, as you read you will see that they show you what they know in other ways. And if Tristan's story is very different than yours, you may still want to explore the effects your own pre-birth and birth have on you today. Keep reading. You might find a piece of your story in the pages to come.

Once you have discovered how your pre-birth and birth experiences are contributing to your present-day challenges, you might feel like there's a mountain of work to climb and your past dictates all there will ever be, that it's the end of the story. Thankfully, challenging early experiences need not define a lifetime if we're taught what to look for.

In the next chapter I will discuss what imprints are and how events in our family's past may affect our own lives, whether that's through parenting patterns that came down from foreparents and affected how our own parents treated us, or through less tangible things. In Chapter 2, I will speak about a unique lens I use to gain understanding about a family's history, called, The Family Field. In Chapter 3, I will discuss easy techniques for communicating with babies and describe how babies commonly communicate with us. In Chapter 4, I explore prebirth events and common challenges with a detailed guide for how to heal those challenges at any age. In Chapter 5, I move on to birth events and common hospital birth interventions, their impact on mother and baby and how to begin to address them. In Chapter six, I write about the less explored territory of miscarriage and twin loss.

CHAPTER 2

The Family Field

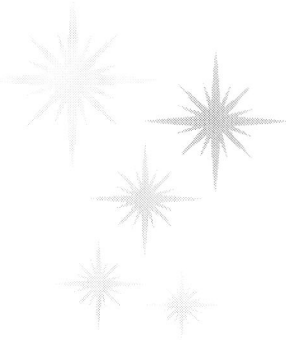

Birth weaves together myriad threads from the past and present. Many of these threads are out of our control, and some of them stretch back many generations. In this chapter I will describe how previous generations can affect life in the womb, birth, and life after birth.

Because this information may be coming to you "after the fact" — certainly after you were born, and possibly after the birth of your baby — be encouraged that it's never too late to heal. I do not want this information to make you feel guilty about not having done all you could for yourself or your child. We live in a world that has not yet fully remembered its connections to forces unseen, so we have to shift our perspective to find them. The information in this chapter is meant to help you understand your own birth and the broader culture of birth more thoroughly, creatively, responsibly, and empathetically. If you find yourself surprised by what you read, don't be too hard on yourself. How pre-birth and birth play out is as much a cultural inheritance as a personal one.

Imprints

We'll begin by looking at how past experiences affect the present, including birth. Nature endows every living being with the ability to absorb and store trauma, though not because it's good to store trauma. Rather, if we want to continue living, we must adapt to the stressful circumstances in our environment. Since life's imperative is life, living beings will choose to live, even in conditions that are not ideal. One of the best ways to do that is to *dissociate*, not fully take in the circumstance, almost as though it's not happening. However, even as we dissociate, a stressful circumstance or shock will leave what is called an *imprint*.

Whenever the charge of an unwelcome event overwhelms our body's ability to discharge the pressure from that event, an injury lingers and doesn't heal. This is an imprint, which in our bodies can take the form of pain or a "dent" in our health. We'll recognize an imprint by our emotional hypersensitivity, our lowered capacity to stay open-hearted during certain triggers, our shame about a certain body part, or our dislike of having that part touched. Perhaps a part of our body will look less healthy or be less engaged. Imprints might also be detected in our thinking. We might have experienced a threat when we were in the womb, during birth, or when we were young. Now, consciously or unconsciously, we anticipate that same threat or one like it. Or there may be other, subtler clues.

The same thing happens to trees, land, animals, and all living things. Well, not exactly the same thing, but all life holds a memory of, and retains the effect of, stressful or incoherent circumstances, and all life can heal with proper attention. The creation of imprints is a normal adaptation to stress and is designed to protect us, if not save our life. Imprints are useful in that they are a storehouse of feelings and awareness that were too much for us to handle at the time. Imagine if we became completely aware of life-threatening circumstances. We might not survive the stress they cause us, never mind the actual event. For this reason, imprints, even if they are bothersome or painful, are actually there as a result of our bodies trying to take care of us.

Take solace. Imprints can be healed. Systems require more energy to sustain incoherence than coherence, so a mysterious mechanism is always moving us towards coherence and integration of imprints. We are offered endless opportunities to notice how challenging events have shaped us. We just need to know what to look for. To begin, examining our Family Field will help us understand some of the imprints that are shaping our present.

Your Family Field

The Family Field model is a way of looking at connections between our own and our family members' past experiences and how they affect the present. The model is based on scientific research into electromagnetic and morphogenetic fields, as well as epigenetics. In order to understand the Family Field, we first need to know what a field is. A field is a sphere of influence, usually invisible, that surrounds living things. For example, the earth has an electromagnetic field around it, as do our bodies. Before we grow a limb in utero, there is a field that shapes how it will grow. These kinds of fields are called *morphogenetic fields*, ones that shape embryos. Morphogenetic fields were widely accepted and used in the first decades of the 20th century by embryologists trying to understand how tissues differentiate to form complex structures like limbs. Today, biologist Rupert Sheldrake talks about how our own body's field interrelates with those of people who have come before us. He calls this *morphic resonance*. The theory of morphic resonance says that physical traits and behaviours of our ancestors will have an influence on how our own traits and behaviours develop. The ancestors who are closest to us, like our parents, exert more influence over us than those more distant.

So how do these fields affect our pre-birth and birth experiences? Picture any kind of field as an invisible and flexible envelope. The envelope is made up of many variables, including the shape of your parents' and grandparents' envelopes; the quality of the air, food, and water around your mother before and while she was conceiving you; the quality of the relationship between your parents; their motivations for bringing you into the world; and the existing cultural climate at the time. Then you come into being with your own envelope, having your own influence on its shape.

The concept of epigenetics, which literally means "upon the genes," is a new way of perceiving what attributes and traits we inherit from our ancestors. Up until only fifteen years ago, traits were thought to come exclusively from genetic inheritance. This meant that people were fascinated with genetic profile and less interested in how the environment of the body shapes organs and therefore people. It's now known that the genes and the environment work together and both are necessary and yet insufficient on their own to create the conditions for development and growth. We come into the world with more genes than we will ever express, and then the environment — which is to say, the world surrounding our family, and our family dynamics — determines which genes turn on and which ones don't. As a result, we appear between the conditions of "nature" and "nurture."

The Family Field model builds on the ideas of morphic resonance and epigenetics to create a lens through which to understand and decode what babies are telling us about the effect of the past on the present. Babies' movements and gestures, and even their unique times of inconsolability, can point out difficulties they experienced during their birth and gestation, and difficulties people in their families experienced before them. For this reason, the Family Field model holds the possibility for healing across space and time. Every new child brings an opportunity to address these objects.

For example, it's common for grandparents or great-grandparents to have come from another country, one in which their family may have lived for several generations or even centuries. The grief they felt at leaving their friends and family, culture, language, and even religion was rarely given the attention it deserved and is still rarely spoken of. You can imagine that arriving on new shores and attempting to assimilate into a new culture were very disruptive, disorienting, and frightening experiences. There may have been difficult travel as they moved from one place to another, and they could have experienced sickness, disease, deaths, rapes, and other horrendous circumstances. Many people have made such moves many times throughout history — whether it was to explore; to escape persecution, disease, or famine; or to pursue new opportunities — and most of them unconsciously brought forward the effects of those traumas (for example, grief, fear, uncertainty), letting them stack up, like plaque, on the bodies and health, of later generations.

I'll use the term "Objects in the Field" to describe the accumulation of specific moments or events that made an indelible impression on parents, or ancestors, and are still resonating in your family and our society today. Objects in the Field are distinct from imprints as they are transmitted through history in families and cultures and are therefore cumulative. Imprints are overwhelming circumstances from an individual's life. If they are not healed, they can add to Objects in the Field.

I call them "Objects" because when we look at a map of collective imprints across a family's lineage, the consistently ungrieved event, and its consequences on later generations, creates a connecting thread between people in that lineage and literally forms a shape or an object on a family map (see Figures 1 to 8). Examples would be the grief never grieved for those people involved in the massive Irish migration during the potato famine; the unacknowledged grief, and the lack of accountability from the Turks, for the deaths of millions of Armenians at the hands of the Ottoman Empire; or the unexpressed grief and lack of accountability for the thousands of women who were forced into organized sex rings in war-torn Yugoslavia. Many of these tragedies and injustices have happened throughout history and are still happening today. When these large-scale cultural events, which radically change the demographic and societal profile of a place, go unseen, publicly unacknowledged, and often, as a consequence, ungrieved, there is a lasting ripple for those living, those to be born, and, I believe, those already dead.

Objects in the Field can also be the legacy of familial violence, sexual abuse, addiction, emotional unavailability — incidents and habits that likely originated in personal hardships, and were fortified by cultural norms. The continual presence of these habits in the Family Field can influence how babies are conceived, how they are born, and how they develop their sense of self. Later we will look at how these same influences persist throughout life and shape behaviour in children and adults.

Your Own Prebirth And Birth's Influence

We, as adults, both male and female, bring children into the world in a way similar to the way in which we were brought. Everything, from how we were thought of before we were conceived to the way we were born and nurtured, shapes our understanding of how things should be. For example, your family may have had a positive view of raising a family, so when you were conceived, you were welcomed into a ready and willing family. Those circumstances continue to shape you today, mentally and physically. Or your parents may have been living in circumstances that challenged their ability to celebrate your arrival and support you along your way. They might have been living with poverty, recent immigration, nutritional deficits, unaddressed sexual or physical abuse, or addictions. Even though it was a long time ago, it is your responsibility as a parent and an adult to become aware of possible influences from your past. You cannot change history, but if you are able to differentiate these past Objects in the Field from your own sense of self, you, or you and your child, can create a future that's more defined by what you want in your life.

Family Field Charts

As you work with the Family Field, you will look back through your first experiences, your parents' early experiences, and, possibly, your ancestors' experiences. You will quickly realize that using this perspective takes the pressure off babies and mothers, who are often seen as exclusively responsible for pre-birth and birth challenges.

Figures 1 to 8 are Family Field charts. The background of every chart is a U-shaped field (Figure 1). The left side of the U is a funnel holding the mother's ancestry. The right side of the U holds the father's ancestry. The bottom of the U is where we see what is happening today. The figure of a child is usually placed there when the chart is filled out.

However, before you, your partner, or your child were conceived, there were already Objects in the Field (Figure 2). Different shapes denote different objects. For example, I use a star to indicate a nicotine or smoking inheritance when someone was in the womb, a light coloured circle for exposure to alcohol, and a darker coloured circle when there's been a major migration in the family history, which likely included leaving loved ones and, depending on the circumstances, could also have included major illnesses or deaths of loved ones along the way. I have even used a darker circle when the parents of a child moved homes or cities during the pregnancy. You can assign shapes relevant to what you know about your inheritance, or you can use my examples and add more when needed. You may want to create a shape that honours abortions, miscarriages, or babies who died in the womb or at birth before you or an ancestor was conceived. Figure 3 shows one possible layout of objects and imprints you and your partner might carry from your Family Fields.

Figure 4 shows how a child sits at the confluence of both funnels and is potentially imprinted by Objects in the Field from each side. All of these experiences belonging to your family will have an influence, especially if they haven't been discussed and have been passed down through the generations. As you gather a composite image of Objects in the Field from your own and your partner's family, you will learn what may be resonating in your or your baby's present-day challenges.

It's worth noting that positive influences are inherited too. They create coherence in a family and in a child. In order to return coherence to what has been incoherent, we seek to articulate ungrieved and unspoken experiences that are suspended in the Family Field.

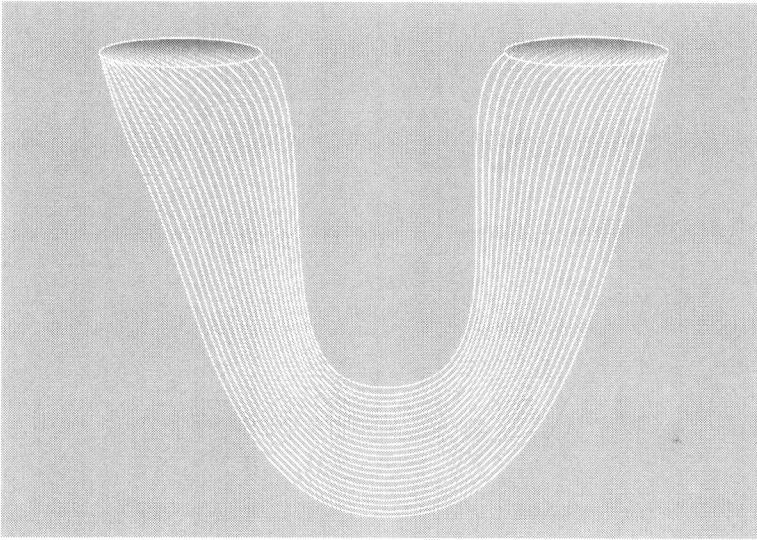

Figure 1: *The unconditioned Family Field.*

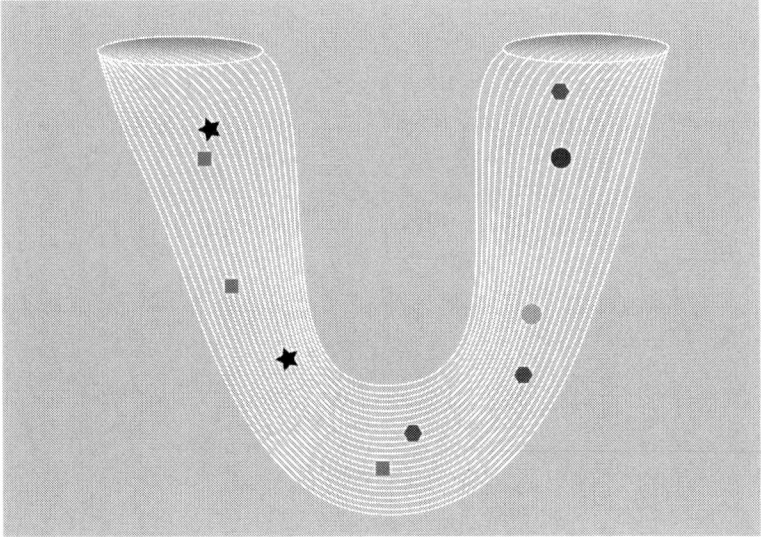

Figure 2: *Objects resonating in the Family Field before conception.*

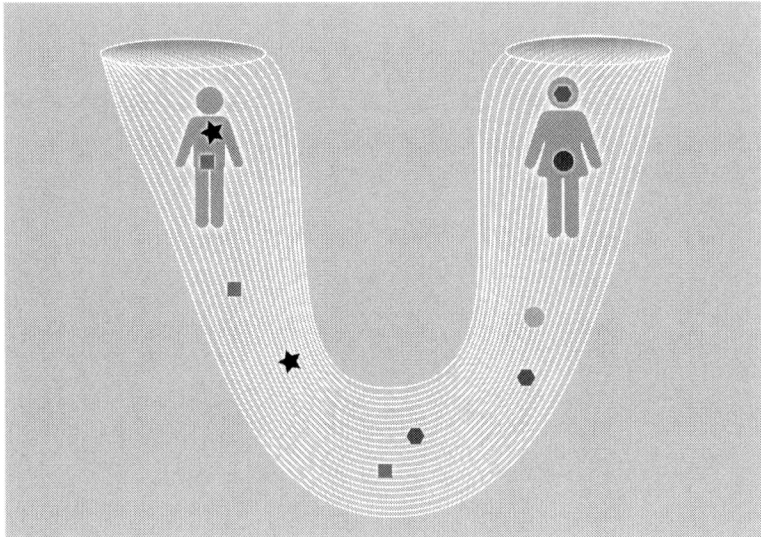

Figure 3: *Objects in the Field with some objects presenting as symptoms in the parents.*

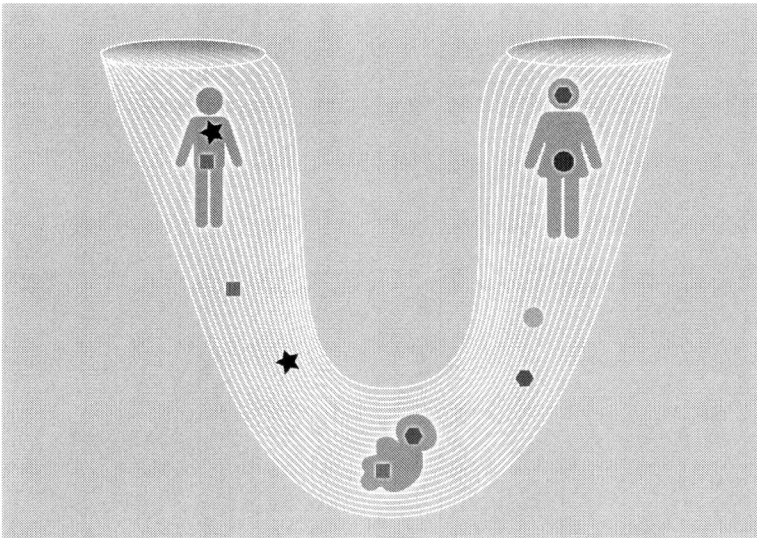

Figure 4: *The next generation resonates with Objects in the Field with latent or expressed symptoms.*

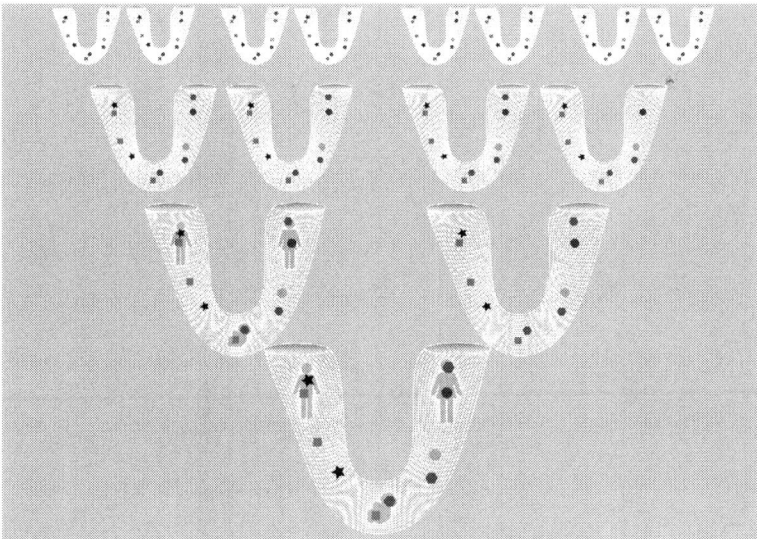

Figure 5: *Family Field chart showing lineages of Objects in the Field.*

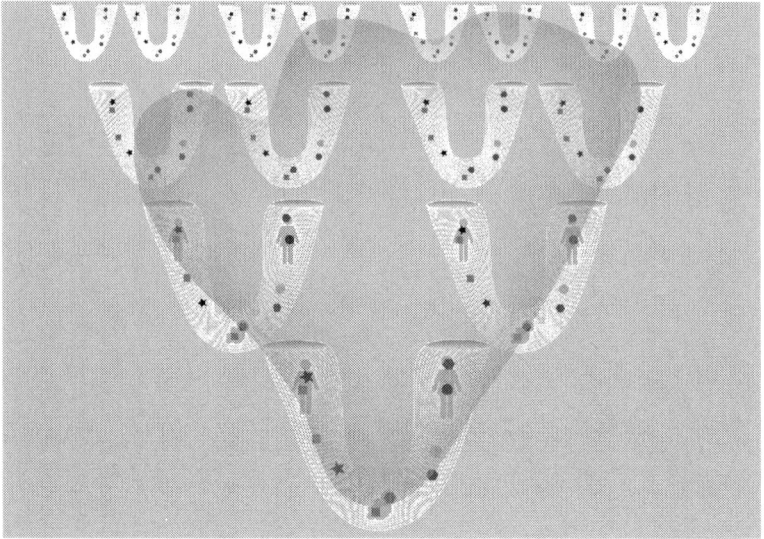

Figure 6: *Links between family members across space and time who share Objects in the Field.*

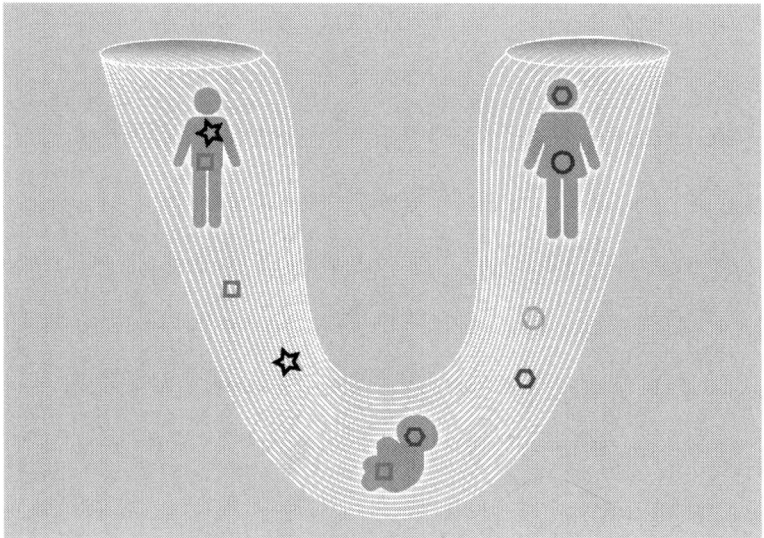

Figure 7: *The clarifying effect of differentiating Objects in the Field. The history of the object stays, but has less influence. Symptoms lessen or disappear.*

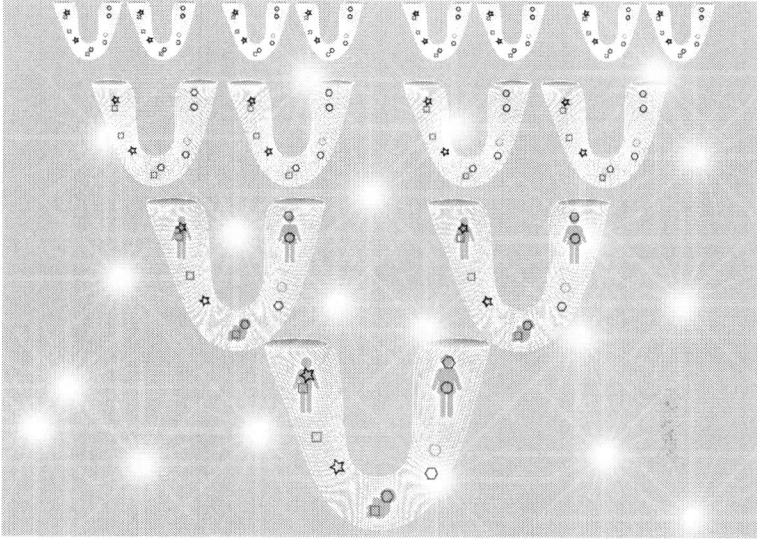

Figure 8: *Differentiating Objects in the Field enhances health and vitality across space and time. More light becomes available between and within all.*

Working with Your Family Field

When you or your baby have a sense of what imprints or Objects in the Field your baby may be expressing, it can be interesting to look at the Family Field as far back through your ancestry as possible. The diagram in Figure 5 shows the same objects repeating throughout the family's lineage. For example, you or your partner may have a relationship to alcohol that has threads reaching back to one of your great-grandparents. That great-grandparent may have been an alcoholic, but it could also be that she was sexually abused and drank to cover up the pain. (In the next section I'll speak about how to find out which ancestors hold a connection to the Objects in the Field affecting you or your baby.) It's also possible that you may not know much about your ancestors' hardships. Families often don't speak of such things. Filling in what you know is a start.

Once you have had a look at how objects have repeated, you could draw a line connecting all family members who may relate to a particular Object in the Field. This produces a pattern or shape that connects all of you (Figure 6) and will help you see how old some of the patterns are, and how they are linked to people who have come before you or your baby.

If you find these diagrams simplistic, know that they are. Their aim is to guide you into a mode of thinking and perceiving that extends beyond what seems obvious. Our lives and the events that shape us are complex, and they are often not as neatly laid out as these diagrams depict.

When I do the healing work for the Family Field, sometimes I concentrate on Object In The Field or on one imprint. I give that shape my attention and compassion. (The body-centered techniques for this work are beyond the scope of this book.) Sometimes I also concentrate on the entire shape connecting members of an ancestry, as depicted in Figure 6, so to hold them and their experiences all at once. When we do the work for ourselves and our children, we change the appearance of those imprints or Objects in the Field (notice the diffused coloration of the objects in Figure 7) and essentially reshape the history that influences the next generation. If families can differentiate and heal what is in their immediate Family Field, I believe it is then possible to untangle and, in a sense, "clear" the objects in the larger Family Field (Figure 8). Notice how all the objects in Figure 8 are colourless and inactive because of the healing that has gone on. The Object in the Field can no longer be sustained, and the essential nature of individuals and entire ancestries radiates. Unwanted history is not forgotten or dismissed after healing; it simply has less influence in the present.

Ancestral Redemption

We, or our children, are the latest buds on a long vine. If we're blessed, that vine is intact. More often, though, the vine has been tangled or severed in places or, for reasons already mentioned, has not thrived. Old cultures have ways of remembering the dead and do so regularly. In technologically advanced societies we sometimes know the names and stories of our ancestors, but often they are people we've never heard of or thought about. Still, it is surprising how many people have an awareness that a dead relative "has been with them," or feel they are "finishing something" for a relative they don't know.

When I'm working with an unsettled baby or child, occasionally an image of an elderly person, who is seemingly from a different time period, comes to my attention. If that happens, I ask the parents if there is an ancestor who might have a connection to what's happening in front of us. I try not to lead with any suggestions of age, appearance, or even gender, so that parents will trust their own instincts. Often the child will relax when the ancestor is discussed. Children are important mirrors for the Family Field, and it's frequently through them that Objects in the Field are revealed. For that reason, babies are some of the most important translators in our societies. Decoding their language is an essential step to restoring humanity where it is missing. The love you give, and the healing you do with, yourself and your babies redeems past, present, and, of course, future generations.

I've given an example of how I inquire about the Object in the Field while working with families. You can also do this for yourself, following these suggestions:

> *Acknowledge a place in your life or in your body that is unsettled. If you are inquiring on behalf of your child, acknowledge what you perceive is incoherent for him or her. With your Family Field drawing in front of you, ask to be shown a constellation, a series of nodes or dots above the funnel that includes you or your and your child. Instinctively place dots or nodes wherever you feel is appropriate. Sit back and look at the shape that forms when you connect all these dots, starting from the one highest above you or your child and moving downwards until the line connecting the dots touches you or your child. Meditate on that line or shape. Indicate to that line or shape, which is your Object in the Field, that you are here to bring coherence to what has been incoherent. Indicate that you are here to give voice, feeling, or movement to what could never be said, felt, or shown before. Hold this intention as you read through this book, occasionally referring back to the dots or nodes you've found on your Family Field. They may be the ancestors still holding the Object in the Field with you.*

The rest of the book focuses on specific imprints from either your own or your baby's pre-birth, birth, or early infancy. Know that working with these imprints can shift Objects in the Field. I encourage you to periodically include your Family Field in your explorations, even though we will not return to working with your maps.

CHAPTER 3

How to Communicate

As you work through this book, you might want to refer to this section often. Babies are communicating their preferences as well as their memories all the time, and the subtle clues they give are not always taught to parents. If you are reading for your own healing as an adult, you might find this section helpful as well. It could be that the baby you once were still longs to communicate some of the things mentioned here.

When a mother holds a baby who is crying inconsolably, she often feels she is doing something wrong, and that is why her baby is crying. However, the baby may be reacting to a drug or procedure administered during birth, or to an ungrieved tragedy in the family's past. Although they are not able to communicate directly with us, babies know what's happening to them and remember their experiences. This includes babies who have just been conceived. But how is this possible when they have no sensory organs yet? Although I cannot offer an explanation for the perception babies that young use, I can affirm that I have worked with countless people who report being affected and imprinted by experiences at this early age — even as they are about to be conceived.

When we are approaching babies in the womb, or looking to heal our experiences from these early times, we are contending with a person's *soul*. Depending on the culture you come from, soul is explained in different ways. For our purposes, I define soul as the whole, already wise, ever-present unique consciousness animating us — at the spark of our conception and at every moment throughout our lives until we die.[1]

Soul appreciates being known. The way we look at children once they are born should include an acknowledgement of their soul. I believe the absence of this acknowledgement is the reason so much child abuse and neglect can go on. It takes generations of unnoticed souls to culminate in a culture that tolerates hurting children. If you have never had your soul celebrated or witnessed, you may not be aware of the beautiful indwelling presence. And if you have never felt your own soul, how would you notice it in another? People whose souls have never been celebrated may feel a sense of injustice that other souls have been recognized and celebrated. It's even possible that practitioners in hospitals may have perpetuated harmful birth practices because they could not bear another child having it better than they did. For these and other reasons, transforming how we treat babies, children, mothers, and our own bodies is vital and requires healing both our personal histories and our cultural inheritances. Looking at a person, no matter their age, with a humble and attuned lens, and with awareness of our own hurts, increases the probability that we will notice and revere their soul. In turn, the quality of presence and honouring that greets souls during pre-birth and birth shapes how those individuals will later view their own selves.

Courting Soul

At the moment of conception, imagine someone else is there, someone carrying the song of your sovereign self, an emissary from the ones behind the veil of what can be seen. And if conception has already happened, even if years have passed, imagine turning to that person, even if it's yourself, and asking them to remember the unique and brilliant self that dwells inside and guides the journey.

Soul is already prominent in pregnancy, especially early pregnancy, and guides the complex movements embryos and fetuses make. I have no way to explain the intelligence of embryos except to suggest they are expressing an intelligence accrued from the experience of all human embryos before them. And the complexity of what they can express would suggest that each embryo's experience exceeds its short life.

The phenomenon of soul guiding movements and gestures does not stop after we are born, but continues all through life. In this book I try to articulate some of the gestures our souls make (through words, postures, movements, and subtler cues) in response to pre-birth and birth.

Rebuilding Trust

You might be surprised to learn that babies can experience betrayal as early as their conception, as they grow in the womb, or at birth. The betrayal could be that they are allowed to suffer a physical injury, or it could simply, although no less profoundly, be the result of an unacknowledged, ungrieved tragedy in that baby's ancestry. Our present health, no matter our age, has roots in many things: our pre-birth and birth experiences; our parents' or ancestors' lives; our physical environment; and, of course, our soul's calling. Babies will naturally avoid situations they don't trust, and if, for reasons of survival, they cannot avoid those situations, they will quietly avoid full connection (dissociation). In this chapter I will explain how parents can rebuild the trust necessary to help their babies dissolve the effects of imprints.

Telegraphing

Babies appreciate finding out what's going to happen before it happens. When we are about to pick them up, change their diapers, or give them a medical test or life-saving surgery, babies appreciate being told about it ahead of time. If we speak slowly and compassionately, explaining what is about to occur, we give their nervous systems an opportunity to adjust, anticipate, and recognize that you, their mother, father, or caregiver, are endorsing what's about to happen.

For example, when you are about to separate from your baby, let her know you will be leaving in a moment. This gives her a choice. Most people don't realize this, but your baby, in her own time, will look away. In a sense, she will be the one to initiate separation. That is the time to move your attention away from her.

If your baby does not look away after you've let her know you are about to end your contact, you can say, *"I see you're not ready yet."* She will hear you, and in time she will look away from you. That is her way of saying, *"Okay, I am ready to break our contact."*

Although you are the parent or caregiver, and it is your job to make sure certain tasks are done for your baby, it is equally true that at times you will have to leave to take care of yourself. Telegraphing helps your baby integrate and accept the upcoming shift, because she gets to participate in how it unfolds. Adults seem to enjoy a little telegraphing too, although they are better able to cope with transitions than babies unless transitions were tough for them as babies.

Giving Space

Try to resist pursuing a baby's gaze. Babies look away when they need a break, either because they're calming down from being excited or because they are managing the charge of an imprint left over in their body from birth or earlier. A baby who has experienced shock during birth or pre-birth will sometimes look away for months.

If your baby is not making eye contact with you or is looking away at something else, know that he is taking care of himself the best way he knows how. Offer yourself as a resource to him by saying something like, *"I see you're looking away, and I just want to let you know that I am here when you're ready. There's no rush. You get to take your time."*

What you're saying is that you understand, you don't need your baby to make you happy, and you are patient and available. This is a subtle but powerful way to help your baby heal any leftover imprints from the challenges of birth or pre-birth.

Do your best not to position yourself in his line of view with the hope that you will lovingly intercept his gaze. He will turn to you when he's ready, and he's best left to do it on his own time in his own way. And who knows? Maybe your baby is enjoying looking at something else. Trust he is doing what is right for him at this time. If he persists in avoiding direct eye contact, you can say, *"I see that you have a feeling that is causing you to look over there and I am over here. Whenever you feel ready, I am here for you."*

You can also explain that you are curious and would like to know what he is feeling. Watch for wriggling, mouth movements, and hand reaching right after you say this. He will start releasing some of the shock in his body by communicating to you with these gestures. Acknowledge that you are seeing these gestures, and encourage him to use you for help any time he wants.

Your desire to have your baby's eye contact is real, but insisting that your baby care for your need to connect through eye contact will make him feel overwhelmed. If your baby is spending most of his time, or what intuitively feels like more than a usual amount of time, looking elsewhere, you might want to do some work with a body-centred therapist — an osteopath, craniosacral therapist, or someone who is skilled working with the body and trauma. Or work back through your baby's and your own birth and pre-natal history, as well as your Family Field, to try to identify what in your own and your baby's timeline your baby might be holding on to. Talk to him about it. Notice what gets your baby's attention, or which story arouses eye contact. Some part of your stories may provoke crying, a significant position change, shuddering, or sounds. Keep the conversation going. We'll go into more detail soon about what could be causing your baby's gestures.

Touch

A parent's heartbeat and body warmth, and the deeply powerful immune and emotional connectors of a mother's milk are powerful healers. Even if a mother is not able to breastfeed because of pain or lack of milk, she should still allow her baby to be near her own and other loved ones' heart, skin to skin. It is through this kind of close touch that a baby comes to know who she is, and a significant amount of pre-birth and birth imprinting can be resolved this way.

The more time a baby spends on her mother's body after birth, the better. In ideal circumstances, your baby decides when she has had enough nursing or when she is ready to separate from the body of her mother or father. Although this type of availability may seem daunting at first, if your baby gets what she needs, she will find tremendous security in her personality and stability in her nervous system. She will naturally grow out of her need for this amount of attachment. You will not raise a "clingy" child; quite the opposite. Babies who are trusted to follow their own needs for contact and feeding have been known to develop deeper self-esteem, better health, and a stronger sense of compassion for the world and people around them.[2]

Touch and connection, essential for life when every baby is born, are even more important for babies whose birth was accompanied by chemicals in the form of anesthetics or contraction augmenters; who were pulled out with instruments in the form of forceps or vacuum; or who were separated from their mothers at birth. All these children will need special care around touch in order to heal. You may find that in this case your baby does not enjoy touch, pulling away or becoming upset when you cuddle her. As heartbreaking as this can be, especially for mothers, this resistance is not because she doesn't want your touch or you; she does, badly. It's that, sadly, touch reminds her of the first kind of touch she experienced while being born — painful touch. In response to her upset, try to remind yourself your baby is having a memory, and it's not because of you. You can use telegraphing here too: let your baby know you're going to touch her before you do, or describe what you're doing: *"That's my hand on your head. Yes, your lovely head. I see that you're shuddering. I'm sorry for what made you feel that way. This is a loving hand and I'm just placing it on your cheek now."* Simply talking about what you're doing can have a very calming and orienting effect on your baby. It is a wonderful way to slow your own nervous system down so you can enjoy the exquisite moment of being with your baby and offering healing.

Attachment Sequencing

Along with touch and telegraphing, there is a helpful exercise you can do with your baby no matter the imprint or object affecting him. *Attachment Sequencing* is an exercise that resembles the movement all mammals make when they leave the womb and make their way to their mother's breast for their first suckle. Right after birth it's called *Self-Attachment*. Ideally, all mammals will have the chance to self-attach, but human babies often miss this important stage of birth because they are brought immediately to the breast or are separated from their mother for a time after birth.

Here's how to do it: Position yourself lying flat on your bed or on the couch. Support your baby by gently holding the bottom of his feet (he will use them to push off you), his back (to support his spine), or his head (let him push gently into your hand and continually give way while staying in contact when he advances into you). As he starts climbing you, from your legs up the front of your body, speak words of encouragement, acknowledgement of what you are seeing him do, and compassion. Your baby will eventually make his way up the front of your body to your breast. Some babies go a little farther, to your shoulder perhaps, especially when they do this with their fathers. That's okay. Your baby may get stuck and cry along the way. If that happens, stop what you're doing, soothe him, and resume again if he isn't too tired. If he is about to overshoot his destination, your breast, then let him know, and he might self-correct.

You can also do Attachment Sequencing in reverse: Start your baby high on your chest, and let him make his way down to one breast with the same gradual motion. If he becomes frustrated or stuck along the way, use the same words of encouragement as you did when he was moving in the other direction.

Attachment Sequencing can be practised three or four times a day. The exercise is an excellent strengthener of your baby's confidence, your bond, and his nervous system. These movements are the first stepping-stones in your baby's later development for creeping, sitting, crawling, standing, and then walking. If Attachment Sequencing is missed in infancy, it's not too late to practice these movements at any age.

Clues to Watch For

As mentioned, babies like to be told what is happening. They also like to be acknowledged, and when you telegraph, you can let your baby know you see what she's telling you about what happened to her. Babies have a way of effectively communicating their suffering. Theirs is a language of *gesture*: movements, sounds, facial expressions, and/or moods that communicate something bigger than what they appear to be. When we're decoding what babies are telling us about their and our pasts, gestures hold an entire story, including where it happened, who was there, what happened, and what feelings are still waiting to come out as a response. The following are some clues about what gestures and noises you'll see and hear your baby make that could lead you to suspect she is remembering something from the past, whether that past is as recent as birth, pregnancy, or conception, or older, from the family's history.

Imprint Crying

Normal and healthy reasons for crying are hunger, frustration, tiredness, physical discomfort, and a soiled diaper. You will notice that when you tend to these basic needs of your crying baby, he'll be consoled and his crying will stop.

In contrast, imprint crying does not resolve when you tend to basic needs. When a baby is remembering an imprint, he is often inconsolable. Something about the present moment reminds him of something troubling from an earlier time, perhaps during birth or even earlier. He may be in pain as he remembers it, or he may be feeling scared. Most likely he has physical and emotional sensations which makes him feel that whatever happened back then is still happening now. It may be that his feelings are a result of an Object in the Field. Taking his feelings seriously has the power to free others who may be affected.

For example, a couple called me because of their baby's colic. No diet change or belly massage could ease his stomach cramps and crying. His parents, who were up with him for hours most nights, were patient but exhausted. During our first treatment, I had the sense this baby was echoing something from an older time, an Object in the Field. I felt this way because there were unclear messages coming from his body. His organs, muscles, and nervous system appeared healthy, but there seemed to be a general overarching incoherence that affected his whole body and even extended beyond his body. I asked his mother how she felt seeing and hearing her son in constant discomfort. I knew she was concerned, but I was listening to the words she might use for a clue into whose tears and discomfort her son was showing.

His mother said, "It reminds me of this lack of confidence I've always struggled with. In fact, my mother had it too, and I sense her mother before her as well."

With that statement, her son's body started moving into positions that signalled he was beginning to release some of the tension. His body curled forward, as though he was back in the womb, and then arched backwards. A new quality was present, one that was coherent, and the coherence was naturally guiding his body along trajectories that could free him from what now looked like an Object in the Field. These various movements went on for another twenty minutes before his body came to rest in a very relaxed position. His eyes were bright and he was lovingly looking at his parents, both of whom were amazed at the process.

While their child was releasing the Object in the Field from his body, each parent also gleaned their own insights. His mother began to feel a sense of confidence in her mothering; his father was thinking lovingly and appreciatively of his own mother, who lived far away. The three of them had regained some coherence, and more love and appreciation, just by perceiving their son's symptoms through the Family Field lens!

Imprint Movements and Posture

Babies attempt to dispel the charge of their imprints by moving and posturing. Because of their imprints' connection to Objects in the Field, they will also try to express those. From here forward, I will focus specifically on how to release imprints but not Objects in the Field. It is possibly that Objects in the Field will resolve while working with imprints, but, as mentioned, a thorough discussion of work in this area goes beyond the scope of this book.

Babies will move into positions reminiscent of the one they were in at the moment an imprint was created.[3] For example, a baby who became stuck during delivery will reenact the position of her "stuckness" when she nurses by getting frustrated and unlatching midway through and crying. Later, stuckness may show up as frustration and discomfort when she meets a challenge while playing or when she attempts to complete a task. Although it won't happen every time your baby or child is reminded of the imprint, the position will often be accompanied by crying or visible frustration. Your baby will even look "stuck." Mothers often recognize their babies' position and intuitively know which moment they are reenacting. After all, mothers and babies were both there when the stuckness or other challenge happened. When babies have the opportunity to release the charge of the imprint, perhaps through Attachment Sequencing, mothers often experience relief as well. Or if mothers are able to release the charge, their babies feel relief.

Children and adults also demonstrate imprint movements and postures. Because adults don't have words for what they remember from their time in the womb and at birth, they will exhibit the same interruptions in their movement or show their imprints in the position they sleep in. People also retain physical evidence of challenging birth experiences in their head, a phenomenon called cranial molding.[4] For example, someone who lingered for a long time getting ready for birth to begin, just at the entrance of his mother's pelvis, will have a certain shape to his head. The same is true if there was a long period of waiting at the exit of the mother's pelvis. These are just a couple of examples of the sorts of physical traits birth leaves in our bodies. Adults heal no differently than babies. They need supportive hands to push into, encouraging words, and a space of total acceptance and compassion as they find the movements that would have accompanied the birth their bodies wished they could have had.

Imprint Feelings

As you'll read in the chapters on pre-birth and birth imprints, these early experiences can leave a myriad of lasting impressions, ranging from "not feeling real" to "feeling unwelcome." They may also lead to an inability to put down roots or a reluctance to "be here on this planet."[5] Alternatively, babies, and later children and adults, may feel they are too slow or that they are being rushed. They may feel unsafe (in a life-or-death way), numb or disconnected, in a fog, stuck, or afraid of choking or being "cut off." Feelings arising from imprints range from kinesthetic — "It feels like I can't breathe" — to emotional — "I feel really bad, really dead." Babies can't express their feelings in words, so they will use crying and movements. Adults, when regressed in therapy, will often have words, but they are sometimes hard to speak.

When approaching imprint feelings in babies, begin a conversation, even if you're not sure what you're seeing. Try saying something like *"I'm not sure exactly what you're feeling, but I'm thinking you seem frustrated, upset, angry, or scared and I want you to know I am here and I am listening, and you can tell me what you need to tell me."* It may take practice to trust that your baby understands you. When you do this, however, you will be surprised by her response. Even better, she will let you know if your instincts were right. Your baby will often stare right at you with wide-open eyes if your compassion is palpable. Crying or discomfort will most likely continue if your baby is in pain or if her present need has not been understood yet. You need not be a mind reader. You just need to be willing to relax and be curious about what your baby is showing you. The more genuine curiosity and compassion you can feel, the more likely it is that your baby will share her emotions with you and settle down.

Imprint Retaliation (Violence)

The most commonly misunderstood communications babies and young children make are hitting and clawing. Understandably, you don't want your baby or child to develop a habit of hurting himself or others. If you have ever been the recipient of a baby's or child's hitting or clawing, you know it can hurt and may naturally provoke your own feelings of hurt, anger, or violence.

When babies and children do this, they are showing you what one of their early experiences felt like to them. They are showing you that something came at them hard and fast, and it hurt. Sometimes instead of showing you on their own body, they'll show you on yours. Showing you what it felt like for them is the best way to tell their story. They have a need to tell this story repeatedly so someone can understand what happened. For babies' bodies to develop and bond the way Nature intended and designed them to do, they require someone to know, show empathy, and demonstrate the kind of protective behaviour they wished for the first time.

The next time your baby or a child shows you a deliberate gesture that causes you pain or discomfort, try wondering what the gesture is saying. You can even wonder aloud: *"Oh… I see,"* slowly or emphatically, *"this is what it was like for you! Thank you for showing me. I'm so glad I know now. I know how it feels for you because I can feel how it hurts me too. I don't like how it feels so you must not have either. Is there another way for you to show me?"*

In one scenario, your child will stop what he is doing and look straight at you with his eyes wide open, as if to say *"Oh! You get it?!"* He may feel understood, and your understanding may be enough to help him stop forever. Alternatively, tears may follow your acknowledgment as he now has the chance to experience the grief, frustration, or anger that accompanied the original event. It may take a few days or months for him to work through it. Continue your curiosity for as long as you see the gesture, offering compassion and your heartfelt regret for not knowing sooner, and offer lots of gentle, soothing contact, preferably skin on skin.

In another scenario, your baby or child might continue showing you where it hurt, no matter what you do. Reassure her that you see what she is telling you and can imagine what it must have felt like. Request that she not do it to you because you can feel how it hurts, and let her know that you are so sorry she was hurt in this way. Invite her to tell you more at any time, and make it clear that you really want to know and understand. Sometimes it takes weeks or even months before the message that you "get it" sinks in. You may need to play a game in which you demonstrate a stuffed animal beating up on another stuffed animal, with you coming in to protect the one being hurt. An older baby or young child may find this settling because it presents you as trustworthy and protective. Seeing another creature, even a pretend one, being hurt is less stressful for your baby than having the memory herself.

Communicating with babies in their own language takes practice. Once you become more accustomed to it, though, the closeness your communication affords you, the wisdom you can glean, and the enormous joy you feel will make the effort worthwhile!

CASE STUDY: *Charlotte, Peter and Henry*

Charlotte wrote to me explaining that her six-year-old son, Henry, was having challenges with his father, Peter.

During our first meeting she said, "Henry bites and kicks and yells, 'I hate you, get out of here,' at his father, and then turns to me and says, 'I wish Daddy would go away.'"

She also explained that Henry was anxious and had been a poor sleeper, not sleeping through the night until he was four and a half years old.

I spoke on the phone with Peter, who had not been able to leave work for our first meeting, and his sincere concern for Henry's well-being was evident. He was as mystified as Charlotte about why Henry was so angry with him.

During our first session, Henry played with toys and drawings. Sometimes I would ask him if he wanted to show me anything. He would consistently tuck himself into small spaces that he called "the cute place" — behind chairs and in between the furniture. Knowing that sometimes children do this not only as a hide-and-seek game, but also to show us what they remember and are still trying to work out from their birth, I let him know I appreciated him showing me "the cute place."

Sometimes he would say, "I can't get out," so I would help him push his body out to his mom. At other times he would find his way out, but he would be unhappy and want to play "baby" with Charlotte. She explained he did this often and sometimes would interfere when Charlotte was nursing his baby sister.

During one particular session, Henry was in "the cute place" and attempting to find his way out when suddenly, out of nowhere, he shouted, "Something tearing, ripping in three!"

I didn't know what Henry meant by "three," but I knew children use single words or phrases to describe their own experience, or sometimes even the experiences their parents were having, during their pre-birth or birth.

When I had inquired about Henry's birth, Charlotte and Peter shared that when Henry was being born at home, he had something called shoulder dystocia: his shoulder had been stuck during the last stages of pushing, which can be very painful, can cause tearing in mothers, and occasionally injures the baby's shoulder, neck, jaw, and face. In Henry's case, right after he was able to free his shoulder, Charlotte had torn. So perhaps "something tearing" meant Henry was aware of Charlotte's body at the time of his birth. It's also possible that Henry was keenly aware of Charlotte's feelings. Charlotte went on to describe the sequence of events at the end of Henry's birth: "He was born, I tore and felt scared, his cord was cut, and then he was held by his dad while the midwives took care of me. "

A few sessions later, with Peter now joining us, Henry, in his usual fashion, was tucked into "the cute place." He started to find his way out with a little encouragement, and once he was out and near Charlotte, he said, "I was scared! Scared of Daddy. Didn't want to leave Mommy yet! Scared of bad."

It occurred to me then that somehow Henry knew someone in the room was scared (Charlotte, scared of the bad pain she was feeling) and had embodied "scared of bad" as his own feelings, as babies often do. Because all babies just want to rest on their mothers after being born, and *scared of bad* was in the room, and Henry was in his father's arms, he had innocently associated all three feelings with his dad: *scared, bad,* and *not wanting to be apart from Mom*. From this, I suspected that Henry didn't really hate or fear his father, but he had associated scared feelings with his father because it was his father's body he felt first, at the same time he was being imprinted by the pain, fear, and "badness" in the room.

It might sound like a leap to conclude that Henry had associated "scared of bad" with his father just because his father had been holding him during a scary time for Charlotte, but babies will bond rapidly with the chemicals, emotions, people, sounds, sights, and events in the minutes right after birth so they can quickly learn how to get on in the world. This is natural and intelligent adaptation. Whatever is in the mix at that moment becomes their sense of reality. What's important to understand here is how sensitive babies are to the feelings of every person in the room while they are being born. For this reason, birth attendants, parents, and whoever else is present must recognize that they can have great influence.

When I asked Charlotte, Henry, and Peter about this possibility, something got very still and clear in the room. The following week I learned that Henry was no longer having issues with his father. During Henry's final session, he went into the "cute place," birthed himself out almost effortlessly, with no interruptions, and smiled up at his mom.

Imprint Play

Many counselors, psychologists, and psychiatrists use *play therapy*, a milieu in which children, in their natural play, have a chance to use their imagination, along with dolls, toys, colouring, or sandboxes, to express deep feelings they haven't been able to integrate or find words for. However, children don't wait until they're in therapy to do this; they express their feelings in play all the time — with their own toys at home, with their siblings and parents, and with friends in the park or at school.

Because you know what birth looks like, you can watch for birth movements in your baby or child. You also need to know what conception, implantation, and later pre-birth movements look like, so you can watch for them in your baby's, your child's, or your own play. I will describe these movements in the next chapter.

When a baby is older, you might see him express deep feelings in play by casting you in roles that don't seem to fit the moment, or by misrepresenting what is transpiring between the two of you, or between him and others. What he is feeling is both real and imagined, and it is amplified because a combination of things is happening: your child's imprint is being triggered, and the present moment is similar enough to the occasion of his earlier imprint that he is reminded of it. Before telling him he is okay or asking him to stop, consider that he is having a memory, and engage him in a healing opportunity.

Tory's story gives a very clear example of one child's play regarding her birth.

CASE STUDY: *Tracy, Richard and Tory*

Tracy came to me with two-and-a-half-year-old Tory, who since birth had been tilting her head to one side. During our first session, Tory picked up a doll that is built in the shape of a pregnant mother, with a little baby who comes out of a pocket in her belly. As Tory played, she positioned the doll feet first rather than head down to show us how babies get born.

Tracy told me that she had been diagnosed early in the pregnancy with HELLP, a form of pre-eclampsia involving high blood pressure, increased liver enzymes, and lowered platelet count. In some pre and perinatal obstetric circles, HELLP is seen as a stress response to factors in the pregnancy from undiagnosed health issues to unconscious reluctance on the part of the mother.[6]

Late in the pregnancy, Tracy was also diagnosed with a condition called *placenta accreta*, in which the placenta grows so deeply into the uterine wall that it has a hard time letting go during birth without causing hemorrhaging. Usually surgery needs to be performed to prevent excessive blood loss. In some circumstances, the woman's uterus must be removed.

As a result of these conditions, Tory's birth was induced three weeks early to avoid further increase in Tracy's blood pressure and other health complications that can arise. Tory was in a breech position, bottom down, when labour began. In the end, she was delivered by C-section. Tracy was blessed in that her uterus was undamaged by the placenta accreta, so she did not have to have a hysterectomy.

Tory's father, Richard, a very devoted father and husband, was away on business at the time. He had planned to be home in good time for his daughter's birth; no one had anticipated the induction and C-section, or that birth would happen so early.

Now, as I worked on Tory's body with my hands, she repeated the movements with the doll, positioning the baby with her feet coming out of the mother first. I kept saying to her, "Oh, this is what it was like for you. Thank you for showing me."

The baby doll continued to be born feet first until I asked the girl, "Tory, what have you always wished could have happened?"

Tory turned the doll head down, turned to her mother, and asked, "Where's the daddy? Where's the daddy?"

Tracy broke into tears. She had never told Tory that her daddy had missed her birth. His absence had been a terrible heartache for both parents, who had wanted to be together when Tory came into the world.

While Tory spoke to her mother, and Tracy cried, Tory's neck let go in my hands, as did her shoulder.

When people involved in any overwhelming circumstance are not given an environment to grieve in, children will often hold the unacknowledged grief in their bodies, thinking it is theirs. Because babies come into the world unaware that they are separate from their mothers, they often take their mother's feelings and combine them with their own.

Tracy's ability to admit to herself how painful it was to go through such a big experience without her husband — something she had been managing quietly on her own until this session — helped her daughter release long-standing postural changes in her neck.

I didn't see the family again, but typically, in situations like this, the child reclaims her confidence, matures naturally, and has greater access to her curiosity and intelligence. You can imagine how such a release leaves them feeling more comfortable and safer to explore!

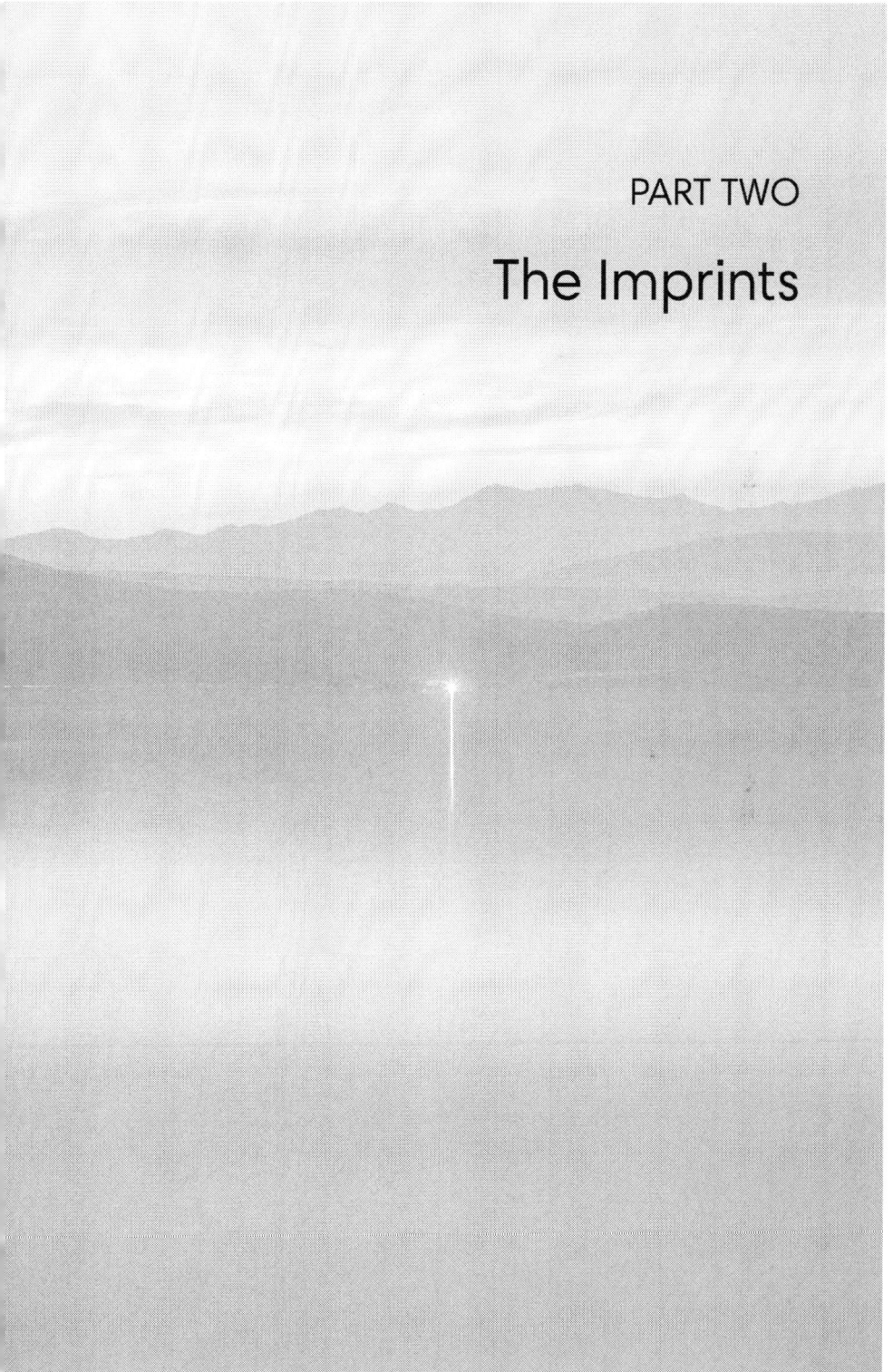

PART TWO

The Imprints

The following observations and recommendations are based on scientific research and clinical experiences involving thousands of people, as well as my own experience involving patients from my clinical work. In no way are these observations and recommendations exhaustive. Use them as guidelines that may offer understanding of your and your baby's experiences.

CHAPTER 4

Pre-Birth Imprints

This chapter takes you deeply into the details of how a baby's experiences, from before conception through conception and the first month of growing in the womb, go on to shape posture, belief systems, and relationship dynamics in infancy and, if left unaddressed, throughout life. The chapter is divided into three chronological subsections: conception or assisted reproduction, implantation, and discovery. Conception is considered the first day or two after lovemaking; implantation is somewhere between four, five, and up to nine days after lovemaking; and discovery is the time parents and the community find out that the baby is present — around two to three weeks after conception when there is no menstruation. Because conception, implantation, and discovery imprints happen during the first month of pregnancy, they can deeply inform the rest of pregnancy, birth, and life.

Early Pregnancy Shapes Birth

It is well known that birth happens in stages. Traditionally, there are three stages: birth starts, birth becomes active, and the baby is born. I add two more stages — the baby's preparation and how she comes to meet her mother — because, as you'll see, they too are important. So in my stages, a baby prepares to be born by dropping further into her mother's pelvis. She initiates birth, and her mother's uterus begins surging. The surges get more intense as the baby travels through her mother's pelvis, turning to pass through the narrowest part of her mother's bone structure. Once through, she is able to exit her mother's pelvis and be born. Finally, she completes birth by gradually making her way to her mother's breast, suckling, and swallowing colostrum (the nutrient-rich precursor to milk) and, if all goes well, after several days, milk.

A baby's preparation for birth will have echoes of how her parents prepared for her conception.[7] *Were* they prepared? Did they perhaps have a "near life experience" where a couple, out of the blue, become aware of the desire to "make" a child, or during lovemaking sense a kind of presence of someone wanting to be with them? Did they conceive her intentionally, or was she a joyful (or regretted) accident? How birth actually begins will recapitulate how her conception went — were her parents intentional, connected to each other, and free of obstacles? Were other influences present at conception? Were there underlying tensions? Was there fighting? You can imagine the many possibilities. The next, more intense, stage of birth recapitulates implantation (how the baby first encounters her mother's endometrium and takes root).[8] Finally, how the baby exits the birth canal and is "born" will recapitulate discovery (how everyone responded upon discovering a new pregnancy was happening).[9] How the parents integrated the news of a baby on the way will shape what happens just after birth, when it's time for mother and baby to meet in the outside world.[10]

"In simple terms, early pregnancy can be seen as pre-exercizing for birth and life," says embryologist Dr. Jaap van der Wal. "What an embryo performs in a morphological way, lends to what a baby expresses at birth and in early childhood physiologically. And what a baby and child pre-exercizes physiologically, lends to how the child later, for example as teenager and young adult expresses psychologically. What a young adult practices psychologically, a mature adult expresses mentally."[11] Dr. van der Wal means that embryological growth is the early education for how our bodies move and grow after birth, and for how we embody psyche and spirit later in life. Another way of saying it: *how your body develops is the early education for how you experience yourself and your relationship to the rest of life.*

It's not hard to see, then, that the first month of pregnancy is critical, yet it is when most people do not know a new life is growing. So as you read this section, be assured it is never too late to revisit and reclaim experiences missed during any of these stages — both for yourself and, if relevant, for your child. The information here will help orient you to what may still be affecting you or your baby, and will also encourage you to give yourself empathy, whether you are the child in question or the parent of a child. As you read, you may find the information challenging. Try to use the challenge as an opportunity to look at what your body is showing you and making you feel. Feelings are an important gateway to healing.

Conception Field

As you'll read in a moment, conception is a pollination rather than a fertilization. For this reason, conception is far more than an egg meeting sperm. Conception is another field, like the Family Field, which is set up long before conception in the quality of the parents' relationship, their health, their Family Fields, and how they feel about welcoming their *conceptus* (a newly conceived child). Consider the conception field to be the context into which a child enters.

A common but mistaken belief is that all children choose their parents. I've met many people who remember feeling reluctant about being born, they felt pushed, or needed encouragement to come here. This is not to say there are mistakes in who finds who, or how parents and their children are paired; it's just a reminder that it's important to avoid rules where mystery is also involved.

Egg Consciousness

An egg is one large cell, full of fluid called cytoplasm. She does not move on her own but is guided by the influences around her. She is open to the unknown, receptive, mutable, and self-supportive. Dr. van der Wal says the egg "lets herself be moved backwards in trust of the future, which phenomenologically could be understood as 'moving backward' in opposition to how sperms move actively forward."[12] Imagine what it feels like to do that!

Eggs are very old in humans. They were produced during the fetal life of the woman. Once a woman is old enough to ovulate, her eggs ripen in clusters. They are thought of as sisters. Although only one or two eggs actually release at ovulation, several mature to the point where any of them could become released eggs. Because only one or two are chosen per cycle, the egg(s) released are privileged; but with that privilege could come a sense of survivor's guilt for the others that did not make it. Even the chosen one, if left on her own for too long, will have a short life. To live longer, she must meet her opposite in the form of a sperm and fuse with one to become a zygote, which is more than a fertilized cell, it is a unicellular organism.

Sperm Consciousness

Compared to an egg, sperm are very young and vital. They were recently produced and live for a few weeks at the most in the epididymis, where if not released, they will be recycled. Sperm are also vying for union with their opposite — an egg. Although the number in one ejaculate can be in the millions, they can be replenished almost immediately. Unlike the egg, sperm are complete, structured and fully realized in their shape. The egg is internally dynamic and more or less chaotic and formless. Sperm architecture, size, and function will never change. You could say that a sperm is already adult in its form and must die to the egg in order to live on in another form. Sperm offer direction, will, and fire to the transformations required if an egg is to grow into a newly forming human. The energy of the sperm also manifests in the headlong burrowing strength an early embryo needs to embed itself in the mother's endometrium a week after conception.

Union

Another common belief is that a sperm "penetrates" the egg's wall, but according to Jaap van der Wal, "no one in science has ever actually seen this."[13] Rather, he says, hundreds of sperm arrive to cluster outside the egg's protective lining, the *corona radiata,* and together they begin to spin for hours. Dr. van der Wal calls this enchanting and science-defying phenomenon the *Preconception Attraction Complex* (PCAC). Imagine that instead of penetration we see a communion, some sort of mystical dance! How accustomed we are to our historical biases, which assume a forceful masculine takeover of the passive feminine? PCAC shows us that forceful and unilateral penetration is not Nature's way. Instead, our assumptions and biases reflect the real and violent histories we all descend from, human-made rather than natural.

The sperms and egg are courting each other, and it's possible that by spinning they are even causing a *transmutation*, where each loses their former self to create a new relationship. On film, the PCAC is a gorgeous, majestic image. If we weren't trained to see cells as strictly biological entities, it would appear that this turning cluster is rendering itself visible through a beautiful display, courting the Unseen and the Great Mystery itself, as if to say, "See this place of beauty! We are here, making way for one of yours!"

Stephen Buhner's poem "Semen" speaks to the union:

Semen is Latin,
from a dormant, fertilized,
plant ovum—
a seed.
Men's ejaculate
is chemically more akin
to plant pollen.
See
it is really
more accurate
to call it
mammal pollen.
To call it
semen
is to thrust
an insanity
deep inside our culture
that men plow women
and plant their seed
when, in fact,
what they are doing
is pollinating
flowers.

Now.

Doesn't that change everything between us?

— from *The Taste of Wild Water:*
Poems and Stories Found While Walking in Woods

Only when she is ready (and who knows what really cues her?) the egg opens her walls. First her *zona pellucida* is dissolved, and then a sperm enters her watery inner world. As mentioned, there is no forceful takeover or penetration by the sperm. He lingers with her, they engage in a mysterious dance, and according to a natural timing, she yields to him or them (in the case of two or more). The sperm has joined the egg inside her body. The new being they've made way for has not yet happened. She is still an egg cell even though he is in there, a so-called *pre-zygote*. And then a few hours later, when the nuclei also fuse, a *zygote*, a new embryo, is forming. After the fusion, an internal cell multiplication happens (mitosis) and then a unicellular body sub-organizes into more and more cells. This will go on for another five to six days.

Conception Imprints

Babies

When I am working with individuals therapeutically, I find that their conception experiences consistently seem to inform the centre line of the body. For this and other reasons, we can guess that there is a trajectory of movement as each being comes to reside in their body. As mentioned, it is not fertilization that sparks a new life. Rather, the cells organize a gathering place that is soon entered and animated by what I will call *soul*. If we trace our way backwards along the line of conception imprints I'm about to describe, there is a trail that leads from inside our body to "out there." So we can guess that conception, particularly the arrival of soul, leaves a highway that eventually becomes the vertical axis around which our spinal cords and spines organize. All vertebrates have a spinal column and spinal cord, and transmit life force along this axis. So if you imagine the length of your spine and how your spinal cord sits inside it, you'll have a picture of the highway along which you were conceived, before you had a body.

Because the trajectory of the soul creates the vertical axis of our spinal cords, conception imprints manifest themselves physically in recognizable movements along the spine. You will see them most clearly when a baby is seated. He will pump his body up and down from head to tail, like an accordion.[14] This compressing and decompressing can sometimes be rapid, especially during frustration. He is attempting to discharge the pressure that has compressed his nervous system along his central vertical axis. The pumping motion relieves the pressure or charge left over from the imprint. Babies who do not have a chance to resolve their conception imprint may have tightness and shortening deep inside the length of their back, which will cause lessened stability or flexibility along certain sections of the spine.[15]

Babies will often look away from you. It will seem that something somewhere else has their attention. They might be less relational. This is another manifestation of conception imprints. Imagine if, when you first showed up, people didn't recognize you or greet you, and they didn't make it completely clear that this was where you belonged — not because they were unfriendly but because they didn't realize you wanted to be recognized and greeted, and couldn't imagine you wanted to be reassured that this was where you belonged. In such a case, you might find it hard to recognize that you belonged here, and you'd be looking for the people or places where you did belong. You'd be waiting for that welcome message.

Children

A child who has conception imprints will tolerate less eye contact, just like the babies who look away. She may be reluctant to enter a room with many people in it, and will tend to sit on the perimeter of a group or play alone in the outer areas of play spaces.[16]

Such a child may need extra time to begin tasks. She has to navigate and relive her memory of conception every time she begins any undertaking, small or big. She may be horrified when she makes mistakes, because each time she is learning something, she remembers a challenge around her conception, and therefore her viability. Conception imprints will show in how well a child is able to learn from her mistakes or reflect on how her behaviours affect others. It's possible her sense of her own desires may be influenced by her conception as well.

A child with conception imprints may have compression and tightness along her spine or in her head, and might display an overall malaise or a fear of living life full-out.

Adults

An adult with conception imprints will have the same issues as children. The difference is that he will have developed more ways to hide his discomfort. Being gregariously warm might be one way to overcome the profound shyness of being with strangers. Staying busy with work or other tasks can help ease the discomfort of being seen by others. He may tend to position himself on the edge of rooms or groups.

When he finds himself the centre of attention, or receives praise from a friend or loved one, he may find it difficult to connect the attention to his own personhood because it exposes his feeling that he is "illegitimate" or "not real." He may feel that the person praising him is talking about someone else. Too much attention can shatter or overwhelm his well-formed defenses. He may wonder whether it's right that he was born, or he may feel as though he was adopted or even that he came from another planet. He never really feels part of something; rather, he always feels just a little strange, not fit for the group or job, and conflicted between wanting to fit in and preferring his own company, sometimes to an extreme degree. Paradoxically, he may be extra sensitive to not being taken seriously or not being listened to. The challenge of feeling unimportant is heightened by the presence of conception imprints.

Finally, some adults have such severe compression (or shortening) of the long axis of their bodies that they are chronically tired, depressed, or unwell.[17] The compression of the spinal cord dampens the ability of life to move through the body. No disease is ever the result of one imprint, but conception imprints often cause a person to be less resilient and less able to discharge stresses.

Healing Conception Imprints

When a person at any age is met with a welcoming gesture, combined with acknowledgement of where she holds the stress in her body, whether this is done with words or, ideally, with soft, caring hands, her nervous system will decompress. She will experience a sensation that she is meant to be here and is therefore real. She will find that she has greater flexibility in her body, greater access to her physical energy, and more emotional balance. She will also feel that she is better able to tolerate groups and is more able to welcome positive attention. A belief that she "belongs here" grows.

Even without a trained therapist, it is possible for a child or an adult to begin to dissolve the impact of a conception imprint. Start by inquiring about the intentions surrounding conception. Were the parents willing or reluctant? If they were reluctant, why? Was someone not ready? Were there reasons from the parents' childhood that were in the way? Was someone drinking alcohol that day? That week? Or heavily that month? Was anybody on medications? What about recreational drugs? How about ceremonial medicines? How were the parents connecting at that time? Were they mutually supportive, with a solid commitment to the relationship? Was there coercion? Was lovemaking personal? Did anyone speak to this incoming soul? (If you or your child were conceived through assisted reproduction, or ART, see the section on ART below.)

If You Are Working on Yourself

Even if you can't remember or don't know the details, you can ask your body to tell you. Your body still remembers what is long in the past. Right away you will notice which questions stir something in you. None of these questions may fit your history exactly, but they will put you in closer relationship to what your body knows.

To forge a relationship with your body, try this exercise:

> *Sit quietly. Notice the activity in your mind. Wait for the sights, sounds, and sensations to quiet down. Even if it's hard to trust that the information is going to come to you, you may notice that you are still eager to do your best. Somewhere you know how to do this.*

> *Breathe.*

> *Imagine your body's intelligence. It may come to you in the form of a colour, a thought, a surge of vitality, or perhaps a simple knowing. Acknowledge how your body's intelligence presents itself.*

> *Ask yourself if you're willing to go another step.*

> *If you find you are, explore this next question:*

"My body's intelligence, please show me the conditions around my conception."

Wait, go very slowly, and trust.

You may even feel emotions or non-descript familiar sensations.

No matter what happens, consider the relationship forged and return to this or any other question whenever you wish.

You may have received an answer, or you may be struggling to feel anything at all. It's okay. You are allowed not to know. Chances are, what you do know still has more to say.

If You Are Working on Your Baby

You may be understandably reluctant to consider the conditions of your child's conception. You may find it hard to believe those conditions would have long-lasting effects, and once you reflect, you may not feel proud of the circumstances. Be assured that remembering the conditions of your child's conception is not meant to judge you, but to create more ease and intimacy between you and your child.

Your most important tool is compassion. The trick is that you will first have to experience compassion for yourself in order to feel it for your baby. Even if your answers to the questions about conception are making you realize some new things, you should not be hard on yourself. This is not to say there are no consequences to your new awareness, but regardless of what happened, your child will eagerly respond to you being compassionate, regretful, and tender about what he or she went through, even if it was because of you!

When you're ready, here's an example of how you can approach the conversation:

You know, sweetheart, I'm not sure if I know exactly what it was like for you, but I'm thinking you remember when you first came here. Although I didn't know you were coming [or you can fill in here with the top things you think need addressing], I now am so glad you are here. I feel sadness [or another feeling] and it's my sadness. I'm going to take care of the sadness, and you get to be the baby.

I'm so sorry I missed this magnificent moment, the radiance of your soul coming to this place to be with us. I have no idea what it did to you to go through that, and I so wish I could have been there so you could feel me. I want you to know that you can tell me about it anytime, and I will be here to listen. You are so welcomed here and so wanted [or whatever the truth is]. I can see that you're trying to tell me. I am listening.

You may have other ways of speaking, because you had unique circumstances when you conceived your child. It is important to be honest about what happened. Although it's unnatural to acknowledge the worst things you fear you did, it is even worse for children to have their story "cleaned up." They *do* remember, and they will have feelings about it, and there's a greater chance of repair if you're willing to talk about it honestly and compassionately.

Even if you're still learning to trust what you're seeing, your baby will absolutely notice that you are speaking directly into the heart of his or her experience. Every baby, no matter the age or stage of development, will give you a sign to show you "I feel understood." They will show you by changing what they are doing: they may look right at you and focus on you. Sometimes, when you've really acknowledged a hurt a child has faced, they may break into tears. This is your baby saying, "Yes! You got it!" These are tears that were likely not shown or known the first time.

Continue to talk to your baby with compassion and curiosity. Don't try to shush him or her while you soothe; encourage the baby to tell you, and make it clear that you are listening, that you are sorry. Tell your baby that you are here and that she or he doesn't have to do it alone this time.

If you feel yourself going into your own emotional response, such as sadness or guilt, remember that it is your job to "hold space" for your child. You must put your feelings aside now, but you should seek compassion and support for yourself from another adult. You deserve this opportunity for growth as much as your child does. If you notice that you're feeling hard on yourself, it may be that someone did not sufficiently hold space for you when you were a baby. Parents often don't realize they are projecting their own unrequited response from childhood, and they react with strong emotions in the face of their children's emotions. If this is the case for you, remind yourself that there will be time for you to get the support you need. But your baby's time is not your time.

Lightly touch your baby's head and back. This helps babies reorganize their nervous systems around the new axis of recognition you are offering. All the while, remember that no imprint stands alone throughout life. With your caring intentions you may inadvertently begin to address issues from a later time, like birth, or from earlier times in the Family Field. Trust whatever arises and follow it, always intending to find more coherence.

If You Are Working with an Older Child or Adult

If the "baby" is a child, teenager, or adult, you can approach with similar sentiments: compassion, regret, and encouragement to speak whenever necessary are still the healing tools.

CASE STUDY: *June*

June attended a pre-birth and birth healing workshop. She had been wondering for some time why she wanted to see people less and less often. At the workshop, she remembered her conception, and as she tuned in to the intentions of her mother and her father, she found surprising information. June had the keen sense her mother had conceived June in hopes of "keeping" June's father from turning his attention away from her. When she tuned in to her father, June could feel herself as a ball of light dropping into the world. As she arrived into her parents' field, particularly her father's, she dropped right past him, as though there was no one there to catch her. She called her father's field "*a void,*" and reported, "No one was there and nothing was there." June's conception frightened her and obliterated her sense of self.

She admitted that she often had a hard time feeling as if she was "here," and when people spoke positively to her, she felt like they were talking about someone or something unrelated to her. Because her parents lacked the capacity to connect with or acknowledge her at her conception or afterwards, June had never had the chance to feel like she existed.

Through slow and gentle verbal acknowledgement, the other workshop participants testified to June's existence. Although it was excruciating for June to confront the memories of her conception, she gradually took in the new information and began to understand how she might have felt if her arrival had been intended and welcomed. At first it was intimidating. Soon, though, a kind of radiance shone through her as she began interacting more freely and spontaneously with the others. June's conception was happening again, only this time in a welcoming environment that was equipped to greet her!

Weeks after the workshop, June reported that the attention given to her conception had allowed her to come to know herself as a unique being with her own consciousness firmly anchored in her body. On the way to this joy, she also experienced profound sadness and feelings of rejection for having been allowed to "drop through without being caught" at her original conception. She said that when she had the urge to isolate herself or stay on the fringe of a group, she could now ask herself if this was a memory of her first conception, or if she was choosing from her now more integrated sovereign being.

Even if you are not sure that it is a conception imprint you're dealing with, it never hurts to tell the person involved (whether it is you, your child, or someone unrelated) that they are wanted, and to speak honestly and compassionately about the circumstances of conception.

Assisted Reproduction

Studies involving twenty-five groups of women from all over the world found that, depending on the country, between 3 and 16.7 percent of women in "developed countries" and between 6.9 and 9.3 percent of women in "developing countries" experienced infertility over a twelve-month period.[18] The same study found that 56.1 percent of the women in "developed countries" sought fertility care, and 51.2 percent of the women in "developing countries" sought fertility care. During 2006, the year of the study, those percentages translated into 72.4 million women who experienced infertility and 40.5 million who received medical treatment for infertility. The study's authors noted that their findings reflected lower than average numbers. Even so, these statistics suggest that more than half the women who cannot conceive seek medical support, which includes assisted reproduction therapy (ART). There are also women who can conceive naturally, but choose to conceive without a partner and turn to assisted reproduction to begin their family. There are several forms of ART. One of the preferred methods is Intracytoplasmic Sperm Injection (ICSI).

Because science and medicine have known for about eighty years that pre-birth and birth experiences, including conception, shape our later health and life, I'm going to describe the process of ICSI, pointing out the differences between natural conception and how practitioners of ICSI facilitate conception. This will give you a sense of what memories a child could have of an ART conception.

In an earlier form of ART, known as In Vitro Fertilization (IVF), the practitioner put the mother's egg in a petri dish with at least 200,000 sperms and waited for them to interact naturally. Essentially, this increased the chances of the egg and sperm meeting. In a later version of IVF, thought to be more effective, the practitioner put the sperm in a gel that surrounded the egg and then removed her protective coating, the *corona radiata*, thus decreasing her resistance to sperm. Because an even greater efficiency was desired, ICSI was developed. In this process, the practitioner uses a needle to insert a sperm into the egg's cytoplasm, the fluid, watery middle.

The egg used for ICSI is unripe, in a state before she would naturally choose to receive a sperm. If she is too ripe, the process will not work. This is one of the "profits" of ICSI, that technicians are able to "fertilize" the egg when under normal circumstances the egg and sperm are not able to fuse, as in the case of egg unripeness or sperm immobility. They can be forced to fuse.

The tail of the sperm used for ICSI is cut off to prevent it from moving around. Then the rest of the sperm is taken into a needle, which is pressed through the *zona pellucida* into the egg.

If you watch this process on film, you can see not only the egg's *zona pellucida* resists being punctured, but the egg also holds her outer membrane intact and even buckles her membrane in half to avoid the needle rather than submitting to being torn. Finally, she can no longer resist: the *zona pellucida* is overwhelmed, and the needle punctures the membrane, inserts the sperm into the cytoplasm, and, upon exiting the egg, leaves a scar along the path by which it entered.

What's important to know here is that conception happens before the egg is ready; it happens outside anyone's body; and the egg is torn open against its will. In contrast, during natural fertilization, as you read in the

"Conception Field" section, a courtship takes place between egg and sperm; it takes place according to their own timing; and the egg willingly yields to the sperm's entrance. With ICSI, the PCAC dance is missed. And in normal circumstances, the egg can be selective, she is not a passive target.

Every child is a blessing and if your child was conceived through ART, it's important to wonder aloud with yourself and your child what that might have been like for both the feminine consciousness of the egg and the masculine consciousness of the sperm in your child today, during ICSI as well as during other steps in the process. You could use words like:

> *Dearest, I remember when your body was just starting to harmonize and grow, and I want to let you know that you may have wondered where I/we was/were or where anyone was because you were not inside me yet. I'm not sure how that might have been for you, but I want to let you know that I'm here now, and that it may have been scary or enraging for you. Know that you can come to me anytime and tell me what that was like for you. I would have loved to have been closer to you at that time, and I'm so sorry I wasn't. It wasn't because I didn't want to; it was because it was the only way I knew how to help you come here. I wanted you and loved you that much [or whatever is true about the conception].*

You may also want to speak about the force, the early timing, the scarring, or whatever stood out for you in reading the descriptions of ICSI and IVF procedures.

You may feel that there weren't any imprints from your ICSI or IVF procedure. I understand that you may see any form of ART as one of the biggest blessings of your life. After all, because of that procedure you now have your child with you! There might be a very mixed picture here. I give you the details because that is what happens, and if left unacknowledged it might have a lasting impact.

It is difficult to know what the long-term outcomes will be for people who were conceived outside their mothers' bodies. The union of their father's and mother's lines included force, the machines in a laboratory, and well-meaning technician onlookers. We will know better in about two decades, when more children conceived through ART find themselves as responsible adults in a therapist's office. For now, let's wonder aloud together with them and simply extend our curiosity and compassion so they need not hold their stories on their own until then.

CASE STUDY: *Tina, Jay and Jacob*

Tina and Jay had wanted to have a child for years, yet no child came.

They finally decided to try ART, and because ICSI had the best success rates for women with endometriosis, which Tina suffered from, they chose it.

Tina and Jay waited with anticipation at home while four embryos began to find their way into being. Many other people waited and prayed too, as the couple informed family and friends of the possible miracle that was happening. The day came for Tina's endometrium to be implanted. One embryo was chosen for what they hoped would be a long life, and the other three stayed frozen.

Tina's pregnancy went well. Often births after assisted reproduction can have complications, but Tina's labour and delivery went smoothly too. Jacob was born and everyone celebrated.

During our first session, Jacob slept quietly while Tina told me all about their birth. Although it had "gone well," she had questions about some of the sensations she felt.

One sensation that had stayed with her was an overwhelming pressure. She described it as "machine-like, metal-on-metal," in her hips, pelvis, and legs. Tina had been able to cope with the pain of birth, but these strange sensations were still on her mind, still troubling her.

I listened carefully to her story, trying to hear what my own intuition was telling me. Nothing jumped out at me. I started to work on Tina's body using craniosacral therapy and osteopathic techniques, which benefit every mother after birth. My hands could feel the tension in her pelvis and hips. Something didn't quite feel "done" yet.

I asked Tina what it was like to have me work on her. She said she could feel that intense metallic pressure she had encountered during birth. Then a vivid picture of Jacob's conception flashed into my mind: a time when metal and machine and pressure all came into play.

Because I can't always be sure if my intuitions are pertinent, I asked, "Tina, could this metal-on-metal pressure be something to do with Jacob's conception?"

Tina's tears, and the sudden large release of pressure from her body, told me there might be a connection.

"I think so." Tina exhaled, with fresh but calm bewilderment. "Yes!"

I was stunned, because I had never dreamed that an ICSI conception could translate so eloquently into a mother's (and possibly a birthing child's) physical experience. With enormous gratitude, I thanked Tina for our time and left.

During our second session, Jacob was awake. I noticed his right shoulder and lung felt restricted. (People's tissues will take on various forms of tension, immobility, or lack of tone in response to overwhelming historical circumstances.) As I started to work on the area, Jacob became agitated and eventually began crying loudly. Not wanting to press him too far into overwhelming emotion, I asked Tina to hold him and soothe him. Then I began again, using Tina as an anchor to explore more deeply what was bothering Jacob.

With one hand on his back and one hand on Tina's back, I tried to sense what his shoulder and lung were trying to say. As I got connected to both of them, I happened to look over and see Jacob's facial expression. To my surprise, he looked obstinate, as though he was not going to give himself fully to the cooing and tender sounds and words of his mother. It was evident his body liked it, as he was snuggled into her, but his head and eyes could not agree. They stayed out of it. When I saw this, I wondered aloud to him about what I was seeing, acknowledging that for some reason he wasn't going to agree or give in.

Just as it had during Tina's session, an image of Jacob's conception jumped into my mind. There he was in the dish, in the clinic, with Mom and Dad nowhere in sight. I wasn't completely confident that this was Jacob's reality, but I went ahead and talked to him about it: "Jacob, I see what you're showing me with your head and eyes, and that this is very important to you, something no one has gotten yet. I want to thank you for being so clear about how you feel, and tell you I'm sorry that it made you feel this way. I don't know if this is exactly right, but I heard about how you came into the world, that you were alone in the dish, with the machines, and that maybe you couldn't feel Mom or Dad, and that would have been very scary, saddening, and even enraging to you. I'm so sorry you went through that."

Jacob listened very carefully to what I was saying.

"I want to let you know that even though you couldn't feel them, Mom and Dad were so excited to know you, so yearning to be with you. I even knew about you, though I hadn't met you yet. And if they could have, I'll bet they would have built a tent all around you and lay near you the whole five or six days you were there, just to love you and be near you. The fact that they didn't isn't because you aren't important or that you weren't there, and it's not because they didn't want to; it was that they were not permitted. I can't imagine what that might have been like for you."

Tina was tearing up, and Jacob was still listening with his head averted from the rest of his body's alignment.

Another strong picture hit me.

"And Jacob, I know about the others. I know you have three siblings, who are still back there, and we're not going to forget about them."

With that, out of nowhere, Jacob turned his head to meet the rest of his body and dropped all his weight into Tina's arms. His body completely relaxed.

"Mom and Dad are remembering those ones as well. And the fact that you've come all the way here, even though they haven't, is a big thing. I know you feel them."

As Jacob relaxed into Tina, I was stunned again by the deep awareness babies can have, not only of themselves, but of others. I may never know whether it was devotion, guilt, or simply love Jacob had for his three siblings, but, again, I felt so privileged to have a window into places that need to be acknowledged.

Implantation Field

Implantation happens four to nine days after conception. There's a wide variation in the time frame because a child, now called a *blastocyst*, must negotiate with the mother how and where to connect.

So much has already happened before even connecting with his mother in the days leading up to implantation: a child is finding his place between spirit and matter; he is also discovering where he comes from and how the body he is growing is guided by all who came before him.

Just after conception, a new body of the zygote still looks like an egg, except there are two cells, both mostly liquid. As hours and several days go by, the egg-likeness begins to give way to sperm-likeness. There are now many cells, smaller than the original two, clustering more and more tightly together. This stage of development ends in a cluster of several tens of cells called a *morula*. Every cell is spoken genetically the same as the next, and the body does not know up from down, or left from right.

The continually growing morula is brushed gently down the fallopian tubes. As he approaches his mother's downy, blood-rich endometrium, the morula begins to change. This change is a crossover point, *where living longer will require being in relationship to another.* The intelligent morula guides a number of cells over to one side of the body until two distinct layers of cells line up along one of the inside edges. The morula now has rows of cells lined up along the inside, and an outside layer of cells making up the outer wall. With this crossover step, he is now a *blastocyst.*

In the second week after conception, even though they have not met yet, the blastocyst begins orienting his body to his mother's. The outer cells, or "outer cell mass", will connect with his mother's endometrium. In the "inner cell mass", where the two layers of cells have lined up, they will later on will face "out" and become, among other things, the child's brain, spinal cord, nails, and teeth. The cells that in the future face "in," will become his digestive system and all the organs that support everyday life: gall bladder, liver, lungs, and part of the kidneys.

This step happens around day four to nine after conception, or as mentioned as late as ten days (a stressful stretch), which is as long as the new life can sustain himself on his own. He must now find home in another in order to continue growing. As he turns himself into a blastocyst, he also prepares to take hold and be received by his mother — *to implant.*

Note that it is because morulas and blastocysts can sustain life on their own that assisted reproduction is possible. With ART, all steps described above would have occurred outside the mother's body, in a lab. At this blastocystic stage, the new life must either re-enter the mother's body or be frozen.[19]

The mother's endometrium is a rich, nourishing place for her new embryo to find a home in. Imbued with conscious and unconscious messages about what it is to live in this family, the endometrium signals to the young one even as he approaches. Is there enough nutrition and other supports to help the young one find his way into being? Is now the right time? Is there enough to support this new life?

Just as he did during conception, the blastocyst will sense the degree of his mother's readiness, and will learn how implantation and "taking root" have been done before him. Even though the blastocyst has his own life force and life imperative, he will have to work with the resources and challenges of his environment. He will begin learning more about the world he will belong to through the messages he receives via that endometrium. As well, the abundant blood vessels in the endometrial wall provide the first food and the primary form of love for the eager embryo.

Implantation Imprints

The implantation imprint is created during the second week of life, when it is no longer possible to live on one's own in the mother's fallopian tube or in a petri dish (in the case of ART). *The second week of life requires contact and relationship.* The dynamics that forge the relationship between mother and blastocyst shape how relationships will be done, as well as how home is taken and how nourishment is experienced, far into the future.

Finding a nourishing and welcoming place in the uterine wall is no small task. It is not uncommon for the blastocyst to approach and then reject the mother's endometrial lining six, seven, or more times in an attempt to find a suitable spot to grow.[20] The mother's endometrium may reject the embryo too. Survival depends on the mother's body's willingness to take the blastocyst in, as well as her willingness to accept the father's intentions for having a child.[21] In modern ART, whether the embryo is accepted by the womb is where the bottleneck most often happens. Even after natural conceptions, it is proposed that at least 50 percent of blastocysts fail to implant securely in mothers' uteruses and more recent studies suggest that the number is closer to 80 or 90 percent.[22]

Like conception, implantation is a courtship dance, this time between mother and baby. "It is the baby that makes the mother pregnant," says Dr. Jaap van der Wal, "not the father." The mother's endometrium is welcoming to an embedding baby to the same degree that she feels herself capable of supporting parenthood. My clinical experience, working retrospectively with adults and children, has been that implanting embryos sense their mothers' reluctance or willingness. A mother may very much wish to have a child in her consciousness, but unconsciously, due to the Objects in her Family Field or due to her concerns about other factors, she may transmit her uncertainty that she can support this child the way she wants to or the way the child would like. This raises a question about how babies are born into emotionally impoverished or abusive situations and live, when loving, available parents can go years or a lifetime without conceiving. Not all things can be understood.

After implantation, mother and baby communicate directly for the first time through shared blood, and within the week a cord will connect them, uterus to umbilicus through the baby's placenta. Because this first connection site is established at the young one's navel, implantation imprints often manifest in movements and postures around the baby's stomach and belly button. These can be challenges with eating, digesting, or elimination. Or they can be postural in the case of an arch or twist at the umbilical area. They can be emotional, taking the form of feeling "empty" or "hollow."

Because most women don't know they are pregnant during the implantation phase of gestation, it's common for them to unknowingly ingest or expose themselves to chemicals or physical or emotional circumstances that they might have avoided had they known they were pregnant. This means implantation imprints are also common, though it's important to remember that it is never too late to repair the effect that complicated implantation dynamics have had on you or on your baby.

Babies

Implantation imprints, like conception imprints, show themselves in the body through signature movements and through deeply engrained belief systems that are expressed at first by gestures, and then later, when children are old enough, by language.

As mentioned, implantation imprints will manifest physically around the middle of your baby's torso.[23] She will express what is known in pre- and perinatal psychology as an *umbilical affect*.[24] The movement accompanying an umbilical affect will originate behind her belly button. A baby might be noticeably folded forward or arched back at the waist, or unable to lower her knees away from her body. By throwing her body back, she might move away from you when you're holding her. Implantation imprints may also show up as challenges in feeding or as weight gain.

Parents sometimes confuse an implantation imprint with a normal evolutionary reflex called the *Moro reflex*. The Moro reflex happens when your baby is alarmed or feels herself falling. She will arch her torso and also wave her hands, with a startled look on her face. The Moro reflex disappears when babies are around seven months old.[25] In contrast, an implantation imprint will not go away after seven months and will become a habitual posture. Babies may regularly interrupt their nursing and their sleep with this particular imprint.

Babies first find their core strength by using their mouths, then later by lifting their heads, and eventually by pushing themselves up from a belly-down position with their arms, so delays in these gestures may be related to implantation (and potentially to birth, which we will discuss later).

The digestive system is an integral support to infant core strength and coordinative development, so we must look at how the digestive system is first organized. This involves how the blastocyst first takes food, in the form of mother's blood, at implantation. It also involves history in the Family Field around nourishment and love. Look back to this early stage of pregnancy when attempting to ease challenges with nursing, bonding, posture, and movement.

Children

Implantation imprints in children manifest as food challenges, digestive tract irritations, and possibly as postural misalignments in their torsos. Although lower back postural problems can come from a variety of influences, exploring the implantation period can be helpful in stabilizing your child's digestion, lower back and abdominals, overall strength, and willingness to bond.

It may appear that your child isn't interested in food or is insecure about whether there will be enough food. Some children who keenly sense unspoken issues in the family or the Family Field will not be able to open the insides of their bodies and take in love in the form of nourishment. Forcing food can increase the alarm the child feels. If chemicals, in the form of medications, recreational drugs, alcohol, cigarettes, or other potentially harmful substances, were present in early pregnancy, children may have a hard time taking anything in, including love. They may feel repulsed because they had no choice about what they were ingesting earlier on. What can look like a power struggle around food or affection is actually a child's best attempt to have a choice where choice was lost earlier.

Adults

Implantation imprints will show themselves in adulthood when individuals go out into the world and begin to support themselves independent of parents. People who experienced repeated failed attempts to negotiate implantation may come and go, never really feeling like they've landed. They will appear unable to settle in anywhere or "find roots." It might be hard to tell the difference between a natural youthful inclination towards adventure and change or an implantation imprint. Frequent upheaval in residences, jobs, and relationships may be a healthy search for authenticity or the consequence of hurtful memories from pre-birth.

People who felt the presence of toxic chemicals in the form of toxic emotions or substances may not have the resources to cope with other people's emotions, emotionally charged environments, or their own internal states. As a result, adults who had challenging implantation dynamics will want to get out of environments that remind them of "toxic wombs," even if they aren't toxic.

Although there are many factors at play in human behaviour, when two people with complex implantation dynamics form a relationship, they will be confronted by a rhythm that challenges their ability to take root together in aspects of the home or in the relationship itself.[26]

Healing Implantation Imprints

Much can be achieved by giving some quiet thought to what was happening during the second week after conception. You may require a trained therapist to work with you in order to access these events.

If You Are Working on Yourself

It's helpful to reflect on your *own* implantation, even if it is your child's you're wondering about or even if you don't plan to have children. Begin by creating an atmosphere of curiosity, a willingness to think about something you may never have explored before. As you scan the horizon of possibilities, imagine that a new area opens up, one that contains information about your implantation. Feel into your body, ask where the knowledge about your implantation lives. You may get a feeling or image or words right away. Don't dismiss them, even if they are surprising. Bow to what just came to awareness. Ease it out by saying you believe your body and your intuition.

You may arrive at your answers deductively, by observing how you fit the descriptions of implantation imprints. If you do, hold your assumptions lightly, proceed with open-mindedness. Don't treat the diagnosis as final. Healing can always happen, and many influences can contribute to habits that look like implantation imprints. You are a mosaic, not a final conclusion.

Try saying something like this to yourself:

> *Dear young, young self. You are so small, so wise, just arriving into your body, and have this big job to take root and find nourishment. I can sense you approaching, and what it's like there, nearer mom. I can attune to what you pick up. It's in your body's feelings right now, and in your emotions. You can share what's there with me. I trust you. I'm sorry someone couldn't understand you at the time, but I'm here now. What would you like me to know?*

You may have a flavour of something. It could be vague. If so, that's because it's from a time before you had words and because it hasn't been heard in a long time. Accept the new language as real. Believe in its strange way of communicating with you. Keep going back and asking again as you hold this young, young place in a warm, gentle surrounding — a healthy, nourishing, supportive womb. You may need to ask about what was happening for your mother — was she supported? Was she well fed? What about your mother's mother? Can you feel her? Or other grandparents? Who in your Family Field shows up as you come into contact with the wall of your mother's womb and your ancestry?

If You Are Working on Your Baby

If you are addressing your own child's implantation, try to remember what was happening in *your life* back during the first two weeks of pregnancy.

Do you remember the season? What you were up to? How were you and your partner relating? Perhaps there was no partner. What was your state of mind about pregnancy at that time? What dynamics were going on in your extended family or your community of friends?

Nothing may come to mind, or you may discover some connections you have previously not thought of. Even if you don't remember, what's it like to try to remember? Do you feel open? Does your attention dull? These observations are worthwhile.

You may need several calm and gentle visits before the question softens into answers from your deeper knowing. Whatever implantation dynamics are at play in your child's life, they will rise out of your deep knowing and come as a surprise to you. They may be new, and even if they are painful, they might be refreshing.

Empathy towards yourself is your next step. Once you've offered yourself some empathy, or have spoken to someone who can empathize with you, consider talking to your baby or to yourself as the baby about the implanting. Do your best to tell the truth from your end, adding your compassion and regret while you tell it. Leave room for your baby's perspective too. If you are the parent, it might sound something like this:

> *Dear one, I want to apologize to you for not having my attention on you and your journey as you found your way into my uterus. I imagine it must have been difficult and at times frightening. I am so glad you made that journey. If I could go back to that time, I would talk to you, feel you as you make your way, and make my body open to you as you settle in. I'm so sorry if you missed feeling me, or for what you encountered instead. I was going through [wherever your attention was at the time or your deep feelings regarding being pregnant], though that doesn't change how important it was that you found your way into my body. I am ready for you to be here. Know you can tell me about it anytime.*

Unwanted Children

It is possible that you are not happy your child is here. Or perhaps initially you were unhappy to be pregnant, but now that your child is here, you are very connected to him. Believe me, you are better to be honest with your child than to conceal your reluctance. This doesn't mean you should tell him you wish he wasn't here or he is unwanted. But you could explain that although he is here and has a sovereign right to exist, you are burdened. A powerful point to make is that your child himself is not a burden. The child has no responsibility for your feelings. You might say that these are your feelings and you're going to take care of them by, for example, finding other forms of freedom or getting extra support, depending on your situation, and it's okay for your child to be a baby. It is good to tell the truth in a way that makes clear your concerns are yours and not the responsibility of your baby. Ensure that you are taking care of those concerns and your baby does not need to take care of them for you. Your conversation may sound like one of these examples:

> It's important to me to make sure I have enough money so that I can care for you the way I want to. I am feeling concern because I have not achieved that yet. It's not because of you.

> It's important to me that my body is healthy in a way that best supports your growth. My concern is that I haven't achieved that yet for us. It's not because of you.

> It's important that I get the support I need from my loved ones because I want to support you and care for you. I am concerned that I have not cultivated that yet. It's not because of you.

> It's important that I become the person I want to become, and I'm concerned that I won't do that; it's not at all to do with whether you deserve to be here. You do.

With every concern you have, differentiate what you are concerned about (or were concerned about at that time) from your baby's existence. Reassure your baby that your concern was because of *your* concerns, not because he existed. Remind him he is welcome on this planet, even if you have concerns for yourself about being his parent. If you continue to be unsure of your willingness to parent your child, consider setting up a situation that will support both of you.

You will come up with the words that resonate for you. If nothing feels right at first, try using some of my suggestions and see what happens. They should lead you to your own means of expression.

It is common that the way we feel about our children is an Object in the Field. In other words, it may be that your own implantation was fraught with ambiguity, and the arrival of a new life might provoke the memory belonging to you or your mother or another of your ancestors. Most of this happens outside our awareness until a child's or our own issues draw our attention back to the object. Consider seeking out a professional with whom you can explore the content of your pre-birth and birth. If this is not a possibility, try speaking to the baby you once were in the way I have described above. Treat yourself with the same tenderness, slow pace, and acceptance that you would wish from your parent.

If you believe this is in fact an old pattern, be prepared to welcome and accept whatever feeling comes to you. Accept that your initial attempts may feel contrived. Accept that they may provoke deep feelings of grief or anger or even numbness. Trust that your body and the baby you once were will hear you. Simply focusing loving attention on yourself will have healing outcomes. Don't worry about the pathway. Your being will lead you to what's next.

Discovery: The Third or Fourth Week

Women know they're pregnant as early as conception, and as late as four or five months into pregnancy. Sensitivity to their body is a factor, and whether they expect regular menstruation or not. A pregnancy test may not show the whole picture. Most commonly, a couple knows they are pregnant after a woman's menstruation time is missed and a pregnancy test confirms an embryo has taken a home in her. How the couple responds creates a big impression on the embryo and on the child and adult she becomes. A person's sense of being wanted forms out of this important time. A child's knowledge she is wanted will also be shaped indirectly by all the people near and dear to her parent or parents. Babies read about the world they are joining through their mother: her bloodstream, her energetic signals, and the sounds and movements she experiences all translate into learning for her embryo. If the mother is supported and celebrated, babies feel it. If she is unsupported, they feel that too.

The discovery of a pregnancy intensifies unconscious issues. The issues that existed between the parents, and that affected each parent from their

Family Fields, can come to the fore. Although a mother's body has been responding to her baby for a month or more already, external confirmation she is pregnant means that what was unconscious or subtle is now a reality. The minds of those involved begin thinking ahead, arranging, dreaming. Babies feel this intensity, for better or worse, as more information about their existence and what their existence means.

If a couple has intended to become pregnant and has been talking to their baby throughout the first month, confirmation of pregnancy will feel settling and natural, and a warm flush of oxytocin will move through both the parents' bodies. The baby will experience this and receive another signal that she is welcome.

If the baby is a surprise, the parents will have myriad feelings. Remember that all signals transmit.

Coming into Form and Growing the Middle

At the beginning of the third week, which is often the period of discovery, a whole new experience happens. He is an *embryo*, and his body is organized into two layers. Now he is ready to grow his third layer or better put, dimension, his *middle*.[27] During week two, according to Dr. Jaap van der Wal, a blastocyst is "not yet an individual within the body, but more or less around." Once the middle dimension begins growing, an embryo is now housed by one spiritual impulse that shares the body. At this point the opportunity for there to be two, in the case of identical twins, ends. The heart, blood, and connective tissue all grow out of this newly arising middle dimension. If conception is a time when soul comes into form, you can think of growing the middle dimension as the time when soul *comes into form to stay*, providing a landscape and occasion through which spirit continues informing matter — or, as Dr. van der Wal says, "matter flames up and spirit flames in."[28]

Matter without spirit does not animate, and spirit without matter does not incarnate. Arrival of soul in the "middle" designates the embryo as a locus for a life to take place, an occasion for the marriage of spirit and matter to occur. The spirit's capacity to enjoy these early trajectories gives it a window into the delight of discovering itself in matter. Our souls speak through experiencing the body. When soul is ignored during these stages, there is suffering. No matter our stage of life, three weeks after birth or three days after death, a subtle presence, can be sensed. It is nothing less than orgasmic to encounter spirit breathing life into your body as it takes shape.

What I'm referring to as soul, science calls *morphogenetic fields (introduced in Chapter 2)*.[29] The morphogenetic fields provide a general frame into which matter is guided to take form. The entire time matter is taking form, spirit is animating the form, making it possible. Matter will not grow, shape, or move without spirit. And once sufficient form has been animated, soul can move into the form and inhabit the form with individual uniqueness. This is "middle". The morphogenetic fields can be thought of as the score, the notes on the page, that guide the conductor and symphony as they play "human." The soloist is soul, bringing a unique performance to a shared and somewhat choreographed, but mostly co-created evolving, piece.

Recognizing Discovery Imprints

The conditions in which a child is first discovered tell her how she can expect the world to receive her for the rest of her life. The messages are unique to every situation and commonly organize around these axes:

I am wanted/I am not wanted

My existence causes comfort/My existence causes discomfort

My existence causes confidence, so I exist confidently/My existence causes reluctance, so I exist reluctantly

Babies

Discovery imprints often show up as left- or right-sided postural habits. Ancient healing traditions have long spoken about the left side of the body belonging to the feminine, which includes all the Family Field dynamics of the baby's mother's lineage, women in culture generally, and inherited feminine traits. The right side of the body belongs to the masculine, which includes the Family Field dynamics of the baby's father's lineage, men in culture, and inherited masculine traits.[30] However, I have also seen patterns that defy a strictly right- or left-sided relationship to masculine and feminine. When we talk about the Family Field dynamics of each lineage, we are describing long-held habits and beliefs about men's and women's attitudes towards children, how parenting "should" be done, and what roles exist for boys, girls, men, and women, which could affect either side. In my discussion below I will assume right side is masculine and left feminine, but bear in mind that this is not a hard and fast rule.

Babies with discovery imprints will tend to lean either to the right (if the imprint is from the father's side) or left (the mother's side), usually from their waist. Sometimes the lean will be imperceptible until many years later, after they've begun walking and running. Weight bearing eventually makes subtler, underlying patterns more visible. In the womb they are energetic and invisible except to a very trained practitioner. Right after birth, patterns are slightly more visible because birth has been very physical, solidifying existing patterns into the body. The patterns become a little more visible in early infancy and may appear in habitual head turning or a favouring of one side of the body. A year or two later the habits are even more visible because the whole body is now involved in daily movements.

Discovering these patterns is not about laying blame. Who knows how long certain patterns have been in families and what circumstances first started them. They may have originated from the prevailing cultural beliefs of a certain time in history. Your focus is not on whose fault it is but on finding an entry point to heal the ungrieved past and differentiate it from your own life and the life of your child, first with authentic raw responses and then, if possible, with compassion.

Children

Once children become toddlers and have had some months on their feet, bearing weight and creating postural habits, they may develop the habit of leaning to one side more than the other. When they are scared or frustrated, they may say words about themselves or their situation that somebody said or had in their mind around the time of their discovery. Children may seek constant reassurance that they are wanted, or they may feel insecure when they are left alone. They may have a habit of showing you pictures of themselves, or drawing pictures of themselves and giving them to you. All children do this at times, but notice which of your child's habits tweaks your intuition. When you ask your child what he or she is remembering, notice the choice of words and what position the child's body is in when he or she tells you. If your child slumps or leans to the left or right while speaking or when upset, consider exploring the discovery time.

Adults

Adults may be showing evidence of discovery imprints when they seek constant reassurance that their presence is desired. They will find it hard to believe they are wanted and loved, and charged dynamics will play out around these very innocent needs for reassurance. Some may even have given up hope of feeling wanted and will act as though they need nothing. Risking rejection can be more painful than living a life without fulfilling intimacy. For them, feeling wanted may be a life-or-death issue. They may also have trouble celebrating their achievements or the completion of tasks or projects, because they're not sure if those are wanted or appreciated. Adults may be reluctant to take their place in society because they fear there is no place for them. Depending on the degree to which the parents did not want their child — ranging from feeling the pregnancy was wanted but happened at an inconvenient time to attempting an abortion — adults may feel frightened to make themselves visible, viable, and sustainable in relationships and economically.

What began for them as an energetic imprint or Object in the Field, and grew into a postural habit, now has become an emotional habit. Imprints begin as morphology (cell structure), they become physiology (cell and organ system behaviour). They then mature into the psychology (emotional and mental behaviour) of the person.

It is never too late to re-pattern a discovery imprint. At any age, life can begin to take on greater ease and flow. By the time healing happens in adulthood, all three levels may need be addressed separately, or they might all be addressed by dealing with one stage of development.

Healing Discovery Imprints

The time of discovery tends to hold more guilt for mothers than either conception or implantation. Mothers are often surprised by their conflicted feelings. Even after years of wanting a child, they can discover a multitude of unanticipated feelings, from lacklustre to extreme reluctance. These conflicted feelings interfere with the natural bonding instinct between a mother, her partner, and her baby. Re-patterning this imprint can provide great relief for all, and the act of re-patterning has the effect of separating the reasons for reluctance or conflict from a baby's identity.

If You Are Working on Yourself

If you are the baby in question, this is such a dear moment for you.

Mothers or fathers rarely experience reluctance because of the child's presence. Instead, reluctance is often driven by fear of an unknown future, sometimes exacerbated by a lack of resources. Or the fear could be that something which happened in the past is happening again. Because you were so sensitive at the time of your discovery — rightfully so, as you were learning so much about your world so quickly — you would have taken any negative feelings at that time as something related to you.

In such a situation, try this exercise:

Place yourself in a quiet place and a comfortable position.

Call to mind one, two, or three people who have really understood you or would be willing to deeply understand you.

Seat them around you in your imagination.

Turn to each one of them and nod to them. See them nod back at you.

With your eyes, tell them you are here to stay.

See what their eyes tell you about your being here to stay.

Keep going around, listening to their words, feeling their presences, and seeing their eyes.

See that you are real to them. You came here. Your being is sovereign.

Let yourself experience the feelings that arise when you try this.

Thank each feeling that arises for coming.

You may feel outraged, sad, numb, but it's important to let yourself acknowledge the feelings that come up. You are not betraying anyone by having each feeling. You were so young at the time of discovery; your only job was to delight in your growing body and experience your soul coming into form to stay. You didn't need a lot, but you did need to be acknowledged, celebrated, and welcomed. You don't have to hate your parents because they did not realize this and did not give you what you needed. Healing is about feeding the deep need your soul, and every soul, has for the world to change because you've arrived.

If You Are Working on Your Baby

It's natural to hold feelings of guilt or, unfortunately, even shame if you were not overjoyed at the discovery of your child. Admitting it to yourself and then, ideally, out loud to somebody who holds no negative judgment can be very restorative. The discovery that you are to become a mother or a father can bring with it the whole Family Field of memories, even if the birth is planned. Going from not being a parent to becoming a parent, or becoming a parent again, are significant transitions, requiring empathy.

If you became pregnant and found that you responded in a way that was less than excited, pleased, or warm, it is important to be compassionate with yourself. There was a valid reason for you to feel that way. It's also important to differentiate any surprises or negative feelings you had from the sovereign life of your child.

Fathers also carry unspoken feelings about the moment they discovered their children. If a man is supported to tell the truth about his feelings without being judged, shamed, or ridiculed, he too will have an opportunity to clear a necessary piece in the Family Field. His child will feel it right away. The same is true for partners of the same sex.

The next step is to compassionately retell the story of your discovery of your child, either to yourself or to your child, acknowledging what it must have felt like to be discovered in these circumstances.

Try a version of the following phrases:

> Now that I know you are here, I feel [express what you are feeling].

> You must have sensed that we/I were/was having [doubts, concerns, angst, reluctance] when we/I first discovered you were here.

> I want you to know that the feeling had to do with [describe the reason] and not because of anything you did.

> You are wanted and we/I are/am so [happy that you are here/curious to know you/loving].

For parents, if you are still reluctant after doing this work, prepare yourself to be honest without feeling guilty. Differentiate your reluctance from your baby's right to be here. Talk about what you are doing to help yourself, and make it clear that it is not your baby's responsibility to make things right.

The work of differentiation is no small task. It takes courage to be honest with yourself about how you are feeling.

You or your child has had the courage to continue on despite what may have been an uncertain or difficult beginning. This does not mean that you or the child will be scarred for life. It is never too late to claim the feeling that has been missed, for you or for you and your child.

CASE STUDY: *Scott, Julie and Ellie*

I visited a couple in their home when their baby was eight months in utero. They had called me after an ultrasound revealed their baby was not growing. The mother was on strict bed rest as a result of the ultrasound. Considering the potential gravity of the situation, she was in great spirits — thinking positively instead of looking at the situation as if there was something wrong.

I thought it curious that the baby had chosen this time in her life to get the attention of her health care providers and parents. I met with the couple and asked them some detailed questions about the period of time when their unborn daughter first came into her mother's uterus — I was looking for patterns. I mentioned to the parents that the climate in which a child is conceived often sets a pattern for the quality of events in the first trimester. I went on to describe how the time when their baby was implanting herself into Julie's uterine wall, and the ease or difficulty of this process, would set a sequence pattern for the second trimester, and the reactions they had as parents to discovering the existence of their baby, sometime around a month into the pregnancy, would have a similar effect on how the third trimester played out.

Since we were dealing with a concern in the third trimester, I asked about what had happened when they found out they were pregnant with their daughter.

I learned that Julie and Scott had been a couple for several years. They had just bought a condo together, and had been living there for several months. Scott was secretly planning a romantic engagement for them, but it had to be carefully timed because they both worked full time. During a summer weekend, they travelled with friends to a music festival, and while camping, hanging out, and having fun, they became more relaxed about using birth control. Thinking it was impossible for pregnancy to happen so easily, Scott and Julie went about their next month as they normally would. It wasn't until thirty days later that Julie began to suspect she was pregnant.

When she confirmed she was pregnant, Scott, whose mind was focused on planning their lovely engagement, was caught completely off guard by the news. Feeling overwhelmed, he withdrew. "Withdrew" in his case included avoiding eye contact with Julie, not acknowledging the pregnancy, and feeling "emotionally unavailable."

Julie had been happy when she discovered she was pregnant, and had no reservations about having their child. She was concerned about how Scott would respond, so when he withdrew, she was hurt. To cope with the impact of Scott's withdrawal, she withdrew too. Her own excitement about the pregnancy, and her connection to the baby, were interrupted for a time.

It took Scott two weeks to come out of his emotionally disengaged state. When he finally emerged and reconnected with Julie, he reassured her that he was, of course, so happy and sorry that he withdrew. He explained that it was because all his attention was focused on surprising her with their engagement, and he had been caught off guard.

Although she was relieved, it took another week before Julie's excitement resumed, and she felt comfortable bonding with their tiny baby inside her.

When I met with the couple, Scott described this two-week period of withdrawal as a familiar habit of his that he called a "glitch." Scott shared that he was used to experiencing "glitches" for two weeks, and they would usually resolve on their own.

Now that I knew a little of the background that brought this family to their situation, we were ready to find out more. I asked them both what stories they knew from when they were conceived, their mother's pregnancies with them, and their own births. Julie told us that she was born by cesarean three weeks early. She had been born this way because she and her mother had an Rh blood incompatibility. This meant that if their blood cells mixed, even a little, during labour or birth, her mother's life would be at risk. At the time, cesarean delivery was the safest way to bring Julie into the world.

Scott told us that he was born two weeks late and had always had the feeling he "didn't want to leave" his mother's womb. He had also had a feeling, although he had never been told this, that he "came along more quickly than planned." He remembers his mother telling him, "The day I told your father I was pregnant with you, he became very stressed and withdrew." As Scott reflected on his mother's words, he suggested the possibility that he and his father had never really bonded because of it.

On the surface, Julie and Scott's situation did not seem unusual. Their story even had elements of romantic irony: they wanted to be with each other, and Scott just needed time to adjust to the change in plans. He had their future in mind, but he had been at an earlier stage in the journey, and Julie just wanted reassurance that he would be there for her. When she learned that Scott had withdrawn only because he needed time to adjust, she felt better.

So why was their daughter not growing? And why was I interested in Julie's and Scott's early lives?

I'm sure their daughter was listening as the four of us sat with all the information.

I wondered aloud, "What similarities might exist between how things are happening today compared to how they went when you two first showed up some thirty-five years ago?"

After a few moments, it was Scott who sat up straight in his seat. His eyes opened wide as he let out an almost relieved exhale. "I did what my dad did with me!"

Scott had made the connection! His own father's reaction had imprinted Scott when he was in his mother's womb. Scott had inadvertently done the same thing his whole life, and now he had done it with his daughter! Scott felt empowered and appeared even happy at his realization.

I suggested that later, after I was gone, he talk to his baby and let her know how sorry he was that he had reacted with withdrawal when he discovered her. He could let her know that it wasn't because of her, but because of something he had learned a long time ago.

He understood what I meant. For Scott, knowing he finally had a deep, resonant understanding of the root of his "glitches" was a welcome insight.

It gave him the choice of how to react to future circumstances that overwhelmed him or were "happening more quickly than planned." I was hoping that Scott's ability to differentiate the past from what was happening in the present would be enough for their baby to continue with her precious growth in the last weeks before she would be born.

A week later, with Julie on continued bed rest and no noticeable change in her baby's growth, I showed Scott some simple craniosacral techniques. Together, we performed a gentle session on Julie. We made Julie's comfort our focus and continued talking to their baby, encouraging both of them to remember this feeling of support when they went into the birth. It was a lovely, restful time together.

Both Scott and Julie admitted they enjoyed just resting and being quiet together. Scott confided that he had done some talking and apologizing to their baby over the previous week. Julie said she had continued "holding the possibility of healthiness and safety" for her baby in her mind over the week. Julie's positive and relaxed attitude was encouraging.

Both times I left the couple, I had a strong feeling that their baby was all right. I was glad that they were being supported by the full spectrum of professionals, from their obstetrician and nurses to their friends and families. I even thought they were being well supported by their baby, because she was good at sending messages (although it was never meant to be her job to get her parents' attention)!

A week after the second visit, I received a call from Julie, who was elated. The nurses had measured their baby and, indeed, she was growing again! Julie was released from bed rest. Her relief was evident in her voice.

I was filled with an overwhelming joy and contentment that warmed me all over. I had never doubted their baby's safety, but it was still thrilling to hear the positive news. I was glad the couple could breathe a sigh of relief and ease their minds. I thanked Julie for letting me know and told her how thrilled I was for her. I put down the phone with a big smile on my face.

Later that day, it occurred to me to check how long a period the baby had not grown. I looked at the calendar and realized, to my shock, that it was two weeks! The same length of time Scott's initial "glitch" had lasted when he first discovered Julie was pregnant! The two-week "glitch" sequence that Scott discovered had now spanned three generations: Scott's father, Scott, and his baby. Happily, Scott's bringing the pattern to consciousness might have the effect of ending the pattern in his lineage. This intriguing Family Field observation made me wonder about all the contributing factors that could affect our health.

My interpretation of this family's situation is that because Scott now understood he was telling part of his early story every time he withdrew, he was able to choose how he reacted to events. By realizing he had learned the two-week withdrawal sequence as a baby in the womb, he was able to sincerely differentiate and apologize to *his* baby for inadvertently passing it on to her. By indicating to his baby that his withdrawal was not because of her but was something he had learned from his own father, he was able to decrease the effect the legacy of the two-week withdrawal sequence was having in the Family Field.

Completing the First Month

By the end of the first month of growth, all the major systems have laid their foundations: the heart, lungs, brain, spinal cord, digestive system, kidneys, pancreas, spleen, adrenal glands, thyroid, liver, and gall bladder will have developed in their primary stages.[31] Tremendous momentum is at work as the mother's blood carries nutrients and her own supportive chemicals from inside her brain to her baby. Mothers and fathers find themselves naturally talking to their baby, singing to him, and touching him through the mother's belly. Life changes all around. This is ideal, but it may not always happen.

Pregnancy has the power to naturally deepen the bond between mother and father. If they are well supported by having enough money, healthy food, and a supportive community around them, they may go through a most romantic time (with the help of huge amounts of oxytocin pouring through the mother's body). Thai researchers, after observing how relaxation and a couple's bond affected the development of babies after they were born, recommended that a couple spend as much time as they can together during the first trimester, and that every day the mother be massaged, look at beautiful pictures, and listen to relaxing and uplifting music.[32] They found that besides the mothers enjoying themselves, there was a correlation between their enjoyment and the relaxation it afforded them, and their babies growing more after they were born.

It bears repeating that most parents do not know they are pregnant during the period when most of the pre-birth imprints happen. For this reason, it is paramount to include a review of the first month of pregnancy when confronting health issues at any stage of life. Know that it is never too late to do the work of recovering the pre-birth period, and especially the first month.

Now we will leave the pre-birth period and begin looking at birth.

CHAPTER 5

Birth Imprints

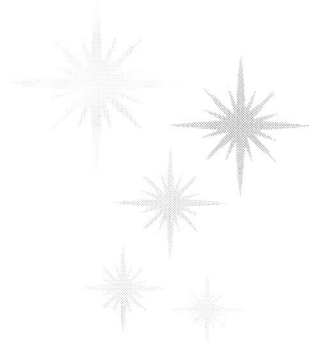

Birth is unpredictable, just like death. There are many kinds of birth and no *right* birth. Every single birth emerges out of the resources and complexities of the Family Field, and even the Family Fields of those in attendance who are not family members. As you've read, the Fields are made up of influences from the past and the present.

Every family can find the resources to prevent Objects in the Field recapitulating at birth. Simply, families can clarify the path of birth by examining their Family Field charts, looking back at their own pre-birth and birth experiences, and exploring what happened during the first month of pregnancy with this child. The present can lovingly include the past, using it for a compass for how to do better. Having the Family Field perspective can make preparation for birth a gentle and loving exploration.

Birth is the time when babies and their mothers will work together most obviously and profoundly. Their ability to cooperate in birth will infuse both of them with the capacity to cooperate well in the future, a skill that will extend to later learnings, projects, and relationships outside their own. Interrupting their innate need to cooperate by either decreasing (with an epidural) or increasing (with induction or augmentation) the action of the mother's uterus will injure the development of this cooperative capacity. These two want and need to work together, and they have all the inbuilt resources to do so. The goal of the people surrounding them is to align with the birthing mother's and baby's abilities, and to support the father as he supports his family. In life-threatening situations we are blessed to have medical interventions like cesarean section, a surgery to open the mother's abdominal wall and uterus to birth a baby quickly. Under non-emergency circumstances, though, the mother and baby will benefit from reverence and support from all those present, as well as reverence and support between all those present.

Resting in the unknown is a difficult proposition for most adults in Western and Northern societies. We are trained from an early age to use our will to achieve outcomes — some people even consider it naïve to trust the natural pace of life. However, any woman who has given birth will tell you that her will, at least until it's time to push, is of no use. No woman can make birth start or make a baby travel faster through her pelvis. Aside from using gravity and breathing and meditating, walking, and praying, birth will go as it will go.

Resting in the unknown is often a quality missing from medical support. The quintessential image of the midwife quietly knitting in the corner while a woman and her baby make their way through birth is not the image we see in televised programs depicting high-adrenaline and high-intervention births. How can birth supporters be encouraged to deal naturally with the very common impasses of birth? How can a mother's feelings of "I can't do this," "I'm going to die," "I want this to stop" be included in the spectrum of normal, if not necessary, stages of a mother birthing? The mother as she has known herself is dying. A new woman is being born as well as a child.

Most mothers and babies experience stuck moments in birth, and there are many ways to overcome the impasse if they don't seem to be able to do it naturally for themselves. Doulas and midwives can speak to the mother, asking her what fears or thoughts she is having to see if they are connected to her early experiences or her Family Field. Ideally, a discussion of the Family Field would occur before labour begins, so if an impasse arises, both mother and doula or midwife already know if it's coming from past experiences, and the birth assistant can remind the mother that she is able to do something different here in the present.

Because birth is so physical, birth supporters can also consider looking at the "high pressure" situation as a form of intense connection. A baby is being squeezed very tightly while making her way through her mother's pelvis and birth canal. There is a reason for this — she is getting ready to move outside the womb. Everything inside her is being awoken to respond to her first contact with gravity. Inside the womb, she has already been touched and been touching for the whole nine months. Her fluids, her placenta, the increasingly tight space of her mother's womb, plus the loving thoughts, sounds, and smells, from her mother and the world around, have all made for connection. During birth, connection, between mother and baby, as well as between people in the room, is necessary. The mother's and baby's hormones, the ones that provide pain support and enough energy to complete birth and nurse, reach peak levels when they are left to do the business of birth. Asking the mother questions or exposing her and the baby to bright lights, the sounds of machines, and another person's stresses (even if they are silent) will only interrupt their natural arc.

Birth and Time

Babies are the ones to initiate birth, and sometimes they initiate birth sooner than planned.

Some babies come early and are called *premature*. These babies often have a wonderful chance to survive the trying condition of being in the world before they're ready because they are gently and sensitively cared for in the neonatal intensive care unit (NICU). I discuss the particular issues these babies deal with at the end of this chapter.

Some babies will have a very premature birth. We call this experience a *miscarriage* or, if it occurs in the sixty days of conception, *early pregnancy loss*. I talk about honouring these babies, in Chapter 6.

Many babies will grow to what we call *full term* or *term* and will likely not need medical support in the form of hospital stays in order to live.

Every family, who intentionally conceives, sets out to have a full-term baby and hopes to have a healthy baby. However, some couples, even before they are pregnant, can anticipate familial medical challenges that are likely to be passed down. Others already know they would like an epidural or a cesarean to avoid pain or to avoid what they believe will cause their vaginas to stretch.

Every decade of the last hundred or more years has seen trends in birth interventions. For example, during the early part of the twentieth century, ether or chloroform, powerful analgesics, were commonly used by obstetricians who thought relief from the suffering of labour was optimal. Inhaling them would render the mother unconscious, protecting her from the pain of birth, and preventing her from interfering with birth — or so it was believed. Later, these gases were replaced by "twilight sleep", a combination of scopolamine (a chemical to supress nausea and other body functinos) and morphine. Their use caused psychotic effects and a complete forgetting that birth had transpired—so much so, mothers were unsure their babies were their own. After twilight sleep was deemed unhealthy for mothers and babies, spinal blocks were used: anesthetic was injected into a woman's spine so she could feel nothing from the waist down. By the 1970s, forceps, calipers used to pull babies out of the womb, were in fashion, and by the 1980s and 1990s, induction, epidural, and cesarean rates started climbing, although they had been in use for many decades already.

Ninety percent of the families I have worked with would call their birth "traumatic" or an event "they experience lasting negative consequences from." These women and babies, and their partners, continue to suffer a form of post-traumatic stress disorder, which can include continued pain, anxiety, a lack of empathy or love for their child and partner, fears something bad will happen to themselves or the baby, low to no libido, decreased energy, sadness, and more.

There is evidence that hospital transfers (transfer from, for example, a home to a hospital or from a rural hospital to a hospital in a major city), inductions, epidurals, augmentations, forceps, vacuums, cesareans, separations after birth, surgeries, and time in the NICU leave an impact even years after the original event occurred. The effects are similar to those experienced by people who suffer from the effects of war, mass migrations, and other trauma.[33] Although some women and their families are given excellent medical treatments for dangerous birth-related medical issues, most are given medical care for non-medical issues, and many families are not told about the challenging after-effects they will live with, caused by the medical treatments that were designed to help them.

Healing Hospital Procedures

The following descriptions of the most common birth interventions at the time of writing move in chronological sequence from those employed during the earliest stages of birth, such as inductions, to those employed in the later stages of birth, such as cesareans and separating babies from their mothers.

Throughout this section, you may be speaking to the child that was you. Taking the role of the child at the same time you are trying to be the good parent is a tall order, but doable.

No experience is irreparable.

Induction

Induction, the artificial early starting of birth can be achieved in two ways. In its milder form, a hormone-infused chemical gel is applied to the mother's cervix, with the hope that the increase in hormones related to birth will stimulate more to come. Mothers often report cramping after the gel is applied to their cervix, and that is often enough to initiate birth. If the gel fails to be enough, the more aggressive version of induction — an IV drip or injection of pitocin, a synthetic form of the birth hormone oxytocin — may be offered. Sometimes there are medical emergencies, high blood pressure, or a condition called pre-eclampsia, that mean birth *must* start immediately. At other times, induction is recommended simply because the mother and baby are considered to be more than ten days past the date they were expected to birth. The calculations of "due dates" are not always accurate, so induction, in the absence of a medical emergency, overrides the natural timing of mother and baby.

An important issue to consider is the relationship of *exogenous hormones* to *endogenous hormones*. The word "exogenous" means "manufactured out-side the body." An IV drip, for example, is manufactured in a lab, outside the mother's body. When hormones are administered exogenously, they do not blend in harmoniously with the body; they may act alone, without the other endogenous (naturally occurring) hormones and chemicals that gen-erally accompany natural birth. For example, in a natural birth, when en-dogenous hormones are secreted, mothers experience a companion rising of endorphins and opiates that allows them to tolerate pain alongside the ever-increasing intensity of birth.

The Effects

Mothers who have been given oxytocin from an exogenous source say it's like being in a boat tossed by the waves of a storm. At first they are in the boat, and the waves are high. After attempting to keep up with the intensity of the storm, with some waves splashing unpredictably into the boat from all sides, the mothers are tossed out of the boat and into the sea. As they try to keep their head above water, and fight to catch their breath and recover from one wave, another wave crashes down before they've had a chance to take a full breath.

A lot of women report that the intensity and the speed of labour after they are given an IV augmentation is more than they can keep up with. Endogenous oxytocin will also create intense surges, but because it's combined with natural endorphins and opiates, these women find it possible to stay in the boat and ride the waves, rather than having the waves crash down over the boat. These mothers are in sync with their bodies.

Babies have the sense of being in the boat with their mothers. With induction, the babies also experience the chaos of being unable to contend with the waves. The boat, naturally designed to carry baby and mother, is overturned, and neither can feel the other moving in sync with Nature any longer. Maybe they can call out to each other in the waves, and hear each other, but the united movement they are designed to share is not available, and they are left to survive the intense, disorganized waves alone.

Most women I know who've had labour induced have decided they "needed" an epidural so they could deal with the intensity of the induction. The full effect of an epidural will be explored next, but, briefly, both mothers and babies experience the combined effect of disharmonious waves from the induction and numbness from the epidural. The induction speeds them up and the epidural slows them down. It is as if you were driving a car with one foot on the accelerator and one foot on the brake.

This leaves both mothers and babies with a feeling of being stuck in neutral, not sure which way to go. One of the effects that mothers notice about five to six months later is that their babies will express disharmony in their natural rhythms. They may resist their internal cues for sleeping and eating. Children and adults whose birth was induced often have an unusual relationship with timing. They react to feeling rushed by resisting or by insisting on being early. Their contrariness is their best attempt to show others what the induction did to them. When birth is allowed its natural onset, babies are the ones to initiate, with the first rise of hormones emerging from their bodies when they are ready. Missing this opportunity due to induction can result in a profound loss of both volition and connection to their own nature and inner authority.

Even if the induction was medically important or life-saving, mother and baby still lose something. Ideally, instead of struggling to keep their heads above water, they would have surged powerfully together, creating a potent, collaborative, cooperative journey. Doing this together would have formed the ground from which their relationship grew. Instead, they have to continually negotiate the memory of these intrusions as they crop up in their relationship.

Healing for Mothers

Mothers need to have their birth story carefully heard. Compassion for what felt like turbulence that she was contending with, not to mention the interruption to the natural process, can help her dissolve the imprint between herself and her baby. This imprint can actually shape how a mother feels about herself. She may be anxious and unable to rest, and she may even feel reluctant towards her baby. Having someone to talk to will help reassure a mother that she was doing her best, that the way things went were not her fault, and that the symptomatic after-effects are not who she is. The intensity, the inability to keep up, the feeling that she couldn't do it are all normal consequences of induction. Gentle bodywork, in the form of osteopathy or craniosacral therapy, will help a mother release the shock she's carrying from managing the mixed signals in her body during birth. She may eventually need to grieve the feeling of being overwhelmed, the resentment at not being able to move with Nature, and the feeling she missed an opportunity to simply "be" with the natural process of birth.

Healing for Babies

Talking to babies about the induction will help them grieve and integrate the loose ends from their birth. When no one tells them what happened, they may go through life feeling something isn't right and assuming the fault is in them. Once they are told "It's not you, this irritation, this panic that you are late or should be moving faster; it was the circumstances you were in," they will relax and be able to trust their internal cues and rhythms.

But you might wonder how this can work. Babies don't speak yet.

Even though babies don't use words, they understand the feeling behind all words. They even understand the feelings when there are no words. They can tell if the speaker is sincere, hurting, angry, unavailable, faking it, or loving them. Whichever parent speaks to the baby about what happened will first need to have received enough empathy for what they went through that they can turn to the baby and offer the same support. Words similar to this could help:

Dear one, I can't imagine what it might have been like to feel yourself moved into birth before your time, how disappointing or maybe even painful it might have been.

I want to let you know that I'm so sorry for how you must have felt; it pains me to think of you suffering. I can't imagine how frightening it was to not be able to feel me clearly. You may have felt separated, or scared that I was not okay and therefore you were not okay.

I want to let you know that the speeding, the pressure, the pain, they are not who you are. They are what happened to you. I won't ever let that happen again. You can always show me what your timing is.

As a parent, you can speak whatever is in your heart. There is no perfect way to speak or words to say. What is very important is to have compassion in your heart.

Epidural

An epidural is the administration of an anesthetic by catheter through the protective sheath and into the spinal cord of the mother. It is commonly used as an option for pain control during birth. While birthing, mothers may reach a point when the pain is too great, especially in the case of back labour (when the baby is "posterior," with the back of his head facing his mother's spine). The effects of an epidural are rarely spoken of, even though they are used so often, and even though the effects are lasting and felt by both mother and baby.

The Effects

Because the protective sheath around a mother's spinal cord is not designed to open to the outside world, it will respond to the needle the same way it would to an injury to her spinal cord. Her immune system will identify that an unwanted intrusion has happened, that tissue has torn, and that a response is necessary. The immune system is designed to protect, so the response will be to wall off and contain the site. Over months, unless treated, a scar will form in the protective sheath, limiting movement, circulation, and strength locally and in areas higher up in her spinal cord. Women will describe having low back pain after an epidural, but it can also manifest as headaches, overall back and muscular tension, and, in more severe cases, depressed vitality, mood, and health.

Those mothers who always planned to have an epidural may have only physical effects, but others, who planned a natural birth, are left with mental conflict in addition to physical restriction. They may ask themselves, *Did I let myself down? Should I have had the strength to go without?* Of course, every woman will do her best and should never be shamed for her choices. Grieving the loss of a *perfect birth* or *the birth that I wanted* is important, and finding a trusted person who can do that with her will eventually soothe her self-deprecation and sometimes even her physical pain. Even if a mother did not plan to use an epidural, it may still be important for her to appreciate how it helped her get through the birth.

An epidural's effect on babies is important too. Babies and mothers are doing birth together, each pushing against the other, both contributing to the hormonal surges accompanying birth and enabling the next step of birth because of their ability to respond to one another. When the epidural is given, the communication is suddenly broken. They've lost the moment-to-moment dialogue they've been relying on. This can leave a baby with the feeling *I have to do it alone* and *I can't feel me or my mother*. The effect could be even more extreme, because babies who are not able to feel their mother might believe *My mother's dead so I must be dead*. The result of these interruptions in a baby's contact and cooperation with her mother during birth is that babies, children, and, later, adults may be reluctant to do anything alone or with another person, because it might remind them of profound separation.

Healing for Mothers

If mothers haven't already looked at the effect the epidural has had on them since birth, they'll want to receive compassion, and be reminded by someone who loves them that the experience is not who they are. If they can connect with their unique experience — and not with how they were told to feel or how they think they should feel — their symptoms, which could be anything from depression and lingering pain to anxiety or lack of care for the baby, will ease. It is important for them to have body therapy to release the tension that's likely left from the needle. Even though an epidural has a profound impact, it is also, fortunately, very treatable, and women will likely recover fully if they receive emotional care and consistent physical care in the form of craniosacral therapy or osteopathy.

Healing for Babies

After a mother has had the chance to receive compassion for her own experience, she can turn her attention to what her baby experienced. Her baby likely experienced some of what has been described here, and anticipating that is helpful, but all babies will have their own story. If a mother evokes compassion in her own heart before she begins speaking with her baby, she will prepare the ground on which they will come back into communication again. She can use whatever words are natural for her. Some could be:

> *I remember when we were working together, and then everything changed. I know that you were there and felt everything. Even though you couldn't feel me, I want to let you know I was there and I know what happened too.*

Usually at this point in a mother's talk, she may hear her baby start to make noises or become unsettled. She can continue with:

> *I don't know exactly what it was like for you, but I can imagine that it might have been scary to not feel me anymore, and I'm so sorry it may have been that way for you. You may even have felt like you were going to die. I want to let you know that I was there with you, and I am so sorry that I couldn't feel you. I really wanted to.*

And then:

> *I'm okay now, and I can feel you. I can see you.*

She may even want to touch her baby's back in the same place where she had the catheter inserted. *"I can feel you now. This is your body. I can feel you with me."*

Once she has offered compassion and regret to her baby, a mother can gently apply a supportive hand, with just as much pressure as it takes to encourage her child to rest on her hand. She can do this on her child's back, legs, and feet, saying something like *"And if there's ever anything you want to tell me about what it was like for you, I'm here. You can always come to me. I'm listening."* An important last piece might be:

> *You know that numbness, that not being able to feel me or your body, that was the anesthesia that came down between us. It wasn't you. There was nothing you did to make that happen, and it wasn't because of you. This feeling is not who you are.*

You may still feel that the epidural was the best solution for you at that time, in which case you may want to explain that compassionately too.

> *Even though all this happened, I had to do this for myself. And I so regret the cost to you, my love.*

As you'll read in the case study involving Cynthia, Eric, and Ella, a very interesting effect can occur with epidurals. When babies start to use their lower bodies, which is almost right away, they may be reluctant to use their legs. They will not want to push with their feet and wriggle through their hips. It's almost as though they took a map of their mother's nervous system during birth that left out details of full engagement in the lower body. This effect is a testament to the rapid learning and agility of the infant mind and brain and nervous system.

The other aspect I have noticed in babies that have an epidural — or any trauma — is that the baby's eyes may look a bit far away. They are not vivid and clear, or you may see a fog if you look right in the eyes. As mentioned earlier when discussing eye contact, a baby who has felt overwhelmed during birth will tend to look away rather than give direct eye contact. It is important not to chase a baby's eyes in this circumstance. Because the intimacy of connection is too intense for them, and can remind them of their birth imprint, babies look away in order to avoid being overwhelmed. You can say:

> *I see that you are looking over there so you can feel yourself, and that's how you're taking care of yourself. I really respect that. When you're ready I'm here.*

Parents might sit for a few minutes, modelling the idea that there's no rush, that they're available, that they're thankful their baby can do this, and that they understand there are reasons for their baby's behaviour.

Another helpful exercise is to let babies spend a lot of time, up to four hours a day, on their mother's or father's bare skin.

Babies often require more time and effort to recover from epidural than mothers do, but after a tender dialogue, like the one described above, plus craniosacral therapy or osteopathy, babies will live with less effect from the epidural and birth interruption.

CASE STUDY: *Cynthia, Eric and Ella*

I met Cynthia and her daughter, Ella, at a postnatal class when Ella was a few months old. Cynthia expressed a desire to come to me because she noticed a habit Ella had formed: she favoured looking to the right and had to "crank her head" to look up. In addition, over the few days right before we met, Ella had become "quite fussy" and often cried. Cynthia suspected Ella was in pain.

During our sessions I noticed that not only did Ella prefer to look to the right, but she rarely looked to the left. Cynthia and I got down on the floor to play with Ella, and while we were there, with Ella lying on her belly, we noticed Ella was also reluctant to use the whole left side of her body. For some reason, Ella hardly wanted to push using her left leg or reach with her left arm, and if we left her too long on her belly, she became tearful.

I asked Cynthia for details about their birth.

"After receiving an epidural when I was dilated to 8 centimetres," Cynthia told me, "the doctors realized that Ella was rather stuck and facing up. We decided to proceed with a C-section to help her."

As I mentioned earlier, when a baby is "posterior," facing away from her mother's spine, the result can be "back labour," where the mother feels an exceptional amount of pain in her low back and rectum. Babies can be born in this position, but they often get "stuck." In these cases, forceps may be used, or the baby may be delivered by cesarean section. This is not to say that babies can't find their way through without forceps or cesarean, as many midwives and obstetricians know how to turn babies, or babies can turn themselves with the help of very attuned encouragement, or be born facing up. But unless hospital staff or birth attendants are looking for Objects in the Family Field and are skilled at deciphering what the birthing mother and her baby really want or need to help them turn or free themselves from the stuck position, intervention will be the best option.

So why was Ella using only one side of her body? Although we could look at her entire Family Field, I started by looking at what might have happened during her birth.

During Ella's sessions, which later included Eric, Cynthia's husband and Ella's father, it became evident to me that for Ella to make the shift she needed, we would have to recreate a feeling that she missed during her birth. Based on her reluctance to use her legs, I decided to start there. I knew that even before the C-section delivery, the epidural sent Ella a message that discouraged her from using her legs. The epidural meant Cynthia could not feel her own body from the waist down, so Ella learned that *this was normal*. Ella's body copied Cynthia's partially anesthetized lower body like a map.

Why was Ella only affected on her left side? Why not on both sides? Those are good questions, and I discovered, in talking to Cynthia, that the answer might be found in Cynthia's discovery imprints. Cynthia told me that she had been treated reluctantly when she was discovered. Cynthia and Eric both knew they wanted to have children, but Cynthia admitted she had always had mixed feelings. This confused her, because she was so sure she wanted children. We talked about Cynthia's early experiences, which may have caused her reluctance, and I explained how she could differentiate them from Ella's by telling Ella that they were her (Cynthia's) experiences, and not Ella's, and apologizing if Ella had inadvertently picked up reluctance from the generation before.

Ella's left side might also have been affected by the strain on her neck when she was being delivered through Cynthia's abdominal wall.

How did we work with Ella, given all these possibilities?

Because Ella showed such eagerness to use her left side and legs, and such frustration when her attempts failed, we went about supporting her efforts. The challenge for children experiencing delays at any stage of development is that in order to progress, they have to confront the imprint or physical problem that caused the delay in the first place. This requires patience while the child productively struggles for a while. In Ella's case, she became tearful on her belly, not only because she was frustrated, but likely also because she was being asked to do something that birth had not prepared her for. We know she wasn't able to use both her legs to push herself out of her mother's birth canal (a necessary stage that would have stimulated the use of her legs). If she was going to do it now, we were going to have to recreate the circumstances of her pushing off her mother's womb, while also understanding how emotionally and physically painful it was for Ella not to do this at birth. Because we may not realize babies are going through this while being born, it is tricky to discern that this is what they're showing us when they are learning to move or are inconsolable.

To encourage Ella to both grieve safely and learn how to use her body, we employed two techniques: compassionate words and touch.

The messages we conveyed were along the lines of *"I'm so glad you're showing us what it was like for you"* and *"We're so sorry this happened and you were hurting and scared"* and *"We want to let you know that this isn't who you are, Ella, these feelings were things that happened to you, they were the anesthetic."*

To show Ella how she should have experienced her body during labour, we used our hands. Over several sessions (after which Cynthia and Eric continued working with Ella at home), we would place a gentle but firm hand on the sole of Ella's left foot to give her an extra amount of support to push from when lying on her belly. We would also put pressure on Ella's left palm when she seemed challenged to reach, until, in a sense, her hand and arm "woke up" and began pushing and reaching without our help.

In addition to the words and touch we used, I gave Cynthia and Ella craniosacral therapy to release pressure from their bodies.

After a couple of visits, Cynthia let me know that Ella was reaching and pushing more with her left side, and that their empathetic talking with Ella calmed her down more easily.

Cynthia said that she could now detect that sometimes Ella's "crying" sounded more like she was telling them something, that there was a speech-like rhythm to her woeful "ah ah ah."

Once Cynthia and Eric learned to recognize Ella's movements and cries as her best way to tell them what had happened to her, Ella moved on past the challenges from her birth.

Five years later, Cynthia and Eric tell me that Ella is a happy, curious child who is interested in art. I was so grateful to spend the time with them.

Augmentation

Augmentation is the administering of pitocin, a synthetic form of oxytocin, through an IV during birth. It has an effect similar to induction, but is used at a completely different stage of birth, and for different reasons.

Augmentation is used when, in hospital language, "there's a failure to progress," a mother is not "dilating," or "birth has stalled." It's not that augmentation is the only way to stimulate birth, but it's one of the hospital's most effective ways to intensify it. And as with induction, there is a difference between exogenous hormones and endogenous hormones.

Because oxytocin intensifies contractions, birth can progress when it is given to mothers during labour, as long as her cervix continues to dilate. But augmented progression doesn't mean the mother gets the natural pain protection her body produces when they reach those oxytocin levels naturally. The effect is that the contractions feel like they are too much. As in the case of induction, they override the teamwork that occurs when a mother arrives at birth on the cue of her baby, with surges intensifying naturally, and mother and baby feeling and communicating with each other.

The Effects

When birth is intensified chemically exogenously, it is difficult for the mother and baby to feel their synchrony. Rather than riding the waves of labour together, they may feel that one or both of them have fallen out of the boat, with waves crashing down over their heads as they surface from the last one. For more details on the effects of augmentation, see the section on effects of induction.

Healing for Mothers

Augmentation, especially without an epidural, is very intense and might overwhelm a mother to the point that she does not feel she can go through with the birth. Mothers are often left in a state of shock, simply because of the intensity of birth. They need to receive compassion from a friend or therapist as they retell this section of their birth story. Hands-on work in the form of craniosacral therapy or osteopathy will help women integrate the chemicals left in the body from this overwhelming event.

A common scenario is that mothers who have had an epidural, which stalls birth, are then augmented to speed birth up again. As mentioned in the induction section, the combination of epidural and augmentation is equivalent to having one foot on the gas and one foot on the brake, which gets mothers "stuck in neutral." Any woman's body wants to heal and discharge the stress from the chemicals, and it will do so if she is provided a safe and relaxed environment in which to explore her feelings.

Healing for Babies

The effect of augmentation on babies is very similar to the effect of induction. The ripples of the stormy seas will linger in babies and will distract them from sensing what their own rhythm in life is telling them. The mixed signals of the augmentation imprint and their own rhythm make it difficult for them to settle and relax. And if augmentation was combined with an epidural, the baby, child, or adult experiences what their mother experienced: one foot on the gas and one foot on the brake, not knowing how to go forward and, therefore, stalled in neutral.

As a baby becomes a child, he will wish to regain the choice he lost in his natural timing. This may manifest as wanting to be the first or the last one to get up in the morning, or the first or last out of the house or into the car. He will want to either speed up or slow down, to somehow reclaim control where it was lost. His body knows that the best way to repair his birth is to get the choice back. Even with a young baby, waking, sleeping, even latching may habitually be interrupted.

> *For parents, this effect can be agitating, and it may be challenging to accommodate their child's need to control timing. If you find yourself entering into a power struggle around timing with your child, one of the best ways to alleviate the conflict is for you to resist feeling controlled, to acknowledge your baby, child, or teenager might be reacting to something that happened to them while being born, and to congratulate them for regaining choice now. Resisting the power struggle is very important, because engaging in it re-enacts the imprint. You could say something like this to a child who has been augmented: I see that you are wishing to nurse on your terms, or you want to have things a certain way and you're finding your way the way you need to. I want to let you know that I'm so sorry for what happened to you, and I understand what you're trying to make right. I'm so glad that*

you have the choice now, and I'm so sorry you didn't have the choice then. And I just want to offer you another way, to use me for connection. I'm here. No one is rushing you this time, and I'm not going to let that happen again., You have all the time you need. You get to choose your timing this time. That rushing, that braking, that stuck in neutral, that's not who you are, and I see who you are, and I'm here and I'm fine this time, and I'm so sorry.

Babies also benefit from bodywork to help their nervous systems discharge the mismatched rhythms they learned from their birth.

If it was your birth that was augmented, you can speak to the young place in you with the same example I've offered above. Once you get going, you'll find your own words for your experience.

Forceps and Vacuum

For hospitals, forceps and vacuum are trusted ways to deal with a stalled birth. We'll look at a third, cesarean, in a moment.

Forceps are adjustable metal tongs that are applied on either side of a baby's head to pull the baby out of the mother's pelvis and into the world. A vacuum machine is attached to whatever section of a baby's head is presenting first, usually the top, to pull the baby out. Both instruments are used to quicken labour or overcome an impasse in the later stages of birth. Both scenarios leave structural injuries and emotional/psychological leftovers for mother and, especially, baby.

Having been through my own healing from a forceps delivery, I can say with certainty that forceps are as painful for babies as they are for mothers. They also have the strong potential to injure the protective layers of tissue, the meninges, around the baby's brain, as well as other parts of the brain itself. And they interrupt a baby's natural sequencing. As I described in Chapter 4, birth begins when a baby enters her mother's pelvis, continues as she drops further, turning midway through birth, and ends when she is born and eventually makes her way to her mother's breast. Babies benefit by being able to sequence their bodies all the way through birth, uninterrupted. Mothers' bodies long for the same sequence.[34]

Mothers are apt to blame themselves or feel guilt when forceps are used, but it is rarely an idea they came up with on their own. In some cases, forceps may have been used with great skill to prevent a more serious health concern for the baby or mother. Regardless of their use, it is important for babies and mothers to have the opportunity to heal from this experience. Healing often requires craniosacral therapy or osteopathy combined with Attachment Sequencing (described in Chapter 3). Healing may take time, depending on the degree of imprinting. And it is important to remember that underneath the imprint is a baby who still wants to deliver herself by cooperating with her mother's natural rhythmic uterine contractions, the way her body instinctively knows how to do.

The Effects

If forceps were used at the end of birth, chances are a mother's pelvis is very sore. The added pressure of the instrument's stretching and force can leave her with bruising or a tear. The pain may be anal, which can make it hard to have a bowel movement without being reminded of the impact of the forceps. Use of the vacuum is not quite as traumatic for mothers because the vacuum device is usually smaller than her baby's head, so she is not stretched to accommodate it.

Mothers may be left with a feeling of more pain than the average birth, and also remorse that the vacuum or the forceps had to be used. A mother who had a birth in which forceps were used might feel her femininity, her womanhood, her motherhood, and her ability to birth have been diminished. She will benefit from telling her birth story and having someone clearly reassure her that these feelings are not who she is but, rather, what she went through. Mothers are less likely to feel diminished by the use of the vacuum.

Parents may notice marks on the skull of a baby delivered with forceps, depending on where the instruments were positioned. The marks will often look like dents on a baby's temples. If the forceps were positioned asymmetrically, the impressions will be positioned accordingly. Skilled obstetricians will usually center forceps quite evenly and will not pull too hard as they wait for the natural surges to push the baby out. But sometimes forceps are placed and used in a way that causes injury. Ideally, obstetricians will not pull hard once forceps are in place. They will resist using force with a vacuum too.

Forceps compress and torque the structures in a baby's skull. The compression can affect how the baby's jaw, eyes, sinuses, and ears develop and function, as well as affecting their posture all the way down once they start using their arms and legs to move. Cognitive and learning challenges, including irritability, hypersensitivity, and compulsive behaviours, can come from a forceps injury as well.

The vacuum pulls up on a specific spot on a baby's soft skull and stretches all the still very vulnerable tissues underneath and around that spot. Vacuum extraction has the effect of pulling up all that's inside a baby's head — sinuses, brain, palate, and blood vessels — and will leave a trail of strain that reflexively pulls on all the membranes inside the body as far down as the pelvis and arches of the feet.

Because birth gives babies their first impression of what "doing it" looks like, an assisted birth will often cause them to fear "doing it" or to develop the belief that they "can't do it," that they'll "need help being pulled out," that they'll "get stuck doing it," or that they'll "be hurt doing it." "Doing it" could mean anything from completing a task, reaching out to their parents, nursing, making movements of any kind, and, later, playing, completing a game, seeing a challenge through, and following through on homework, relationships, and other responsibilities as they become adults.

As with induction and augmentation, babies delivered with forceps or vacuum lose the chance to determine their own timing for resolving the challenge of birth, a result that is heartbreaking and painful. These babies, as they grow up, will be frustrated and overwhelmed when faced with challenges if they don't receive compassion and treatment that includes the chance to finish their birth the way they always wished to. Parents are well advised to talk with their baby about the lasting effects of a forceps or vacuum birth. Because each baby's positioning and each mother's birth is unique, we can't always know if the use of forceps or vacuum was lifesaving or unnecessary. The good news is that both mothers' and babies' bodies know how to finish birth outside the womb, where the effect of instruments can be diminished.

Healing for Mothers

A mother who has a chance to visit a skilled craniosacral therapist or osteopath might find a lot of relief from those sessions. Her uterus still wants to push her baby out without the use of the instruments, and it may hold on to symptoms or emotional leftovers until her body is encouraged to release the imprint from this interruption of the last stage of birth. A bodyworker will also be able to release any congestion from bruising and any lasting tension from tearing in the case of forceps.

After receiving lots of empathy and an opportunity to tell her birth story, a mother may find she is able to let go of her disappointment, fear, and pain, and begin to accept how birth turned out. Her body will heal once she has this chance.

Healing for Babies

Hands-on care with craniosacral therapy or osteopathy is essential and might be needed over years until the baby can really discharge the pressure of the instruments. Every case is different, and consistent love from parents must be included in babies' healing too.

When you see your baby or child is frustrated or scared, or is holding his or her head, you could respond using words like this:

Wow! So that is what it was like for you. This looks like it must have been so frustrating or scary. You must have felt pain and sadness, and even anger.

Telling babies the story of what happened during the end of birth, when they were stuck and someone decided it would be best to use either forceps or a vacuum to help them out, can be valuable for them. You could also say,

I can't imagine what that was like for you, but I'm guessing it might have been painful, frustrating, and scary. You might have been angry, and I am so sorry. I am so sorry it was like that for you.

After simple phrases like these, babies may indicate with a gesture, a movement, sound, stillness, or eye contact that they are listening. You could continue with:

I wish we could have done it the way we wished for, and we could still do it that way now. You are not the pressure, the vacuum machine, or those forceps.

Babies will often cry when you get close to what they've been feeling. It's important not to hush children or give them soothers. Encourage them to keep telling you, and let them know that you're listening and that you want to know. It's best not to tell babies they're okay when they start crying. This is like telling them that what happened during their birth was okay. Imagine that they are telling you a memory they have, and acknowledge they are attempting to reach you with their cries, with how they touch their head or your head, and even with their obstinacy. If you acknowledge everything you see, you will eventually pick up on the feeling they have beyond words. This will build trust between you for life.

Giving a baby support at his feet and bum, and letting him push against you, helps him find the cooperation and potency to get unstuck that he lacked at birth. By pushing against his strength you mimic the action of the uterus. There will be a moment when the birth looks like it's unfolding; the more you relax, stay grounded, and keep things from moving too quickly, the more you will restore your baby's health and confidence in loving relationships.

Cesarean

A cesarean is a planned or emergency procedure in which a surgical incision is cut through a mother's abdominal muscle wall and uterine wall. Her baby is then pulled out of her uterus through the incision. The cesarean may be performed while a mother is already giving birth, or it may be performed before birth starts if there is an indication of a pending emergency. In both cases there are significant imprints left from the procedure.

The Effects

After a cesarean, mothers feel like they're still pregnant, like they are still waiting to push their baby out, because they and their baby did not have an opportunity to complete every nature-designed step together. In the case of cesarean before labour begins, mothers and babies may not have had the opportunity to begin surges at all. These surges not only guide birth, but also guide how a mother's body resolves being pregnant.

Women can have pain at the incision site, although sometimes enough nerves are cut during the incision that pain only arises when nerves start growing back, which doesn't happen till months later, if ever. Women can also have low back pain after a cesarean because all the abdominal muscles are cut, causing a significant loss of core body stability and strength.

Emotionally, mothers commonly feel remorse that they were not able to experience what birth feels like, and they wish they could have completed it. Mourning this missed experience is valuable. Mothers and their babies have intuitively embedded guidance for how to complete birth together, and a craniosacral therapist or osteopath skilled in birth dynamics can offer the opportunity to explore the end of birth.

Babies born by cesarean miss out on the stimulation of their respiratory and musculoskeletal systems that uterine contractions afford. They also miss an opportunity to experience what it's like to successfully work together with the forces of the world (which in this case take the form of their mother). Birth shows them what to expect from the outside world — Is it welcoming? Comfortable or painful? Can they feel their body or are they numbed? (They may be numbed by anesthetic, but the presence of an anesthetic will be promptly forgotten, and the numbness will instead be absorbed as part of their identity.) Will they learn how to make transitions? What about patience, natural timing, and connection? There's been a loss, but within that loss there is an opportunity to heal.

Some of the feelings babies will have because of being born by cesarean are: *"I can't do it," "I can't do it on my own," "I can't feel myself when I want to do something. I go into a numb, stuck place."* Some children or adults report later *"Not only do I feel like I'm doing it alone, but I feel like I'm going to die."* And it's true that somewhere in the sequence of babies who are born by cesarean, the obstetrician may have perceived a signal — like a drop in heart rate or complications with bleeding, blood pressure, or the placenta — that made it clear this birth had reached a point of life or death.

Babies born by cesarean may have increased body tone and tensed or curled-up hands or feet. Or they may show the opposite condition: a lack of tone, floppy limbs and head, and a propensity to sleep a lot. Both of these responses are healthy, adaptive responses to the stresses that arose during birth. The tense baby may be frustrated and angry. And the baby who is less toned or floppy or flaccid may be dealing with the stresses by avoiding engagement, sleeping a lot, and not being fussy. Often the quiet, sleeping baby is seen as a "good baby," because "good babies don't cry and are easy," but quiet babies often cannot engage their volition because when they tried to assert their will, they were anesthetized.

Healing for Mothers

A good place to begin healing mothers is to confront whatever feelings they have because they were not able to finish birth. Each woman will have a unique perspective. Some women I meet say that they are fine with having had a cesarean; they are thankful their baby is now healthy, or they are grateful the doctors averted a life-or-death situation. Other women lament not having pushed their babies out. Some even take the experience personally and come to believe there is something about them that is inadequate.

After women tell their birth story to someone who really hears it and offers compassion and regret for their situation, which may have included epidural, augmentation, or even induction, they begin to feel better. Telling the story doesn't change what happened, but being offered compassion and regret, and reminders that the circumstances of the birth are not their identity, helps enormously in their healing.

Taking high doses of vitamins E and C, along with other antioxidants, will be good for healing what could become a scar. Mothers are best to take at least 800 IU of vitamin E to help heal the deep layers of tissue.

As women heal, I recommend they do a series of exercises to restore core strength to their body. Doing abdominal exercises can help as well, but sometimes when the abdominal muscles have been ruptured or cut it's more challenging to contract and use the transverse abdominal muscle, the deepest layer of abdominal muscles. Because of this, the habit is to compensate using other muscles. I suggest they find either a pelvic floor physiotherapist or a Pilates instructor who will go slowly and help with their particular needs.

Healing for Babies

Depending on how traumatizing a cesarean birth was for a baby (which can be estimated by the number and degree of interventions that took place), parents may notice a baby has a faraway look in his eyes, or the eyes themselves may appear glossy or foggy. As discussed earlier, this "affect" or leftover is often the result of anesthetic and shock. Even if the anesthetic was necessary so the baby's mother was able to withstand surgery, it's important for you to refer to it when speaking to the baby. And, as already emphasized, if the baby is looking away to manage the trauma, it's best not to pursue eye contact by intruding into the baby's line of view. Here's an example of what you could say:

> *I can see, little one, that your eyes are foggy, but that you're there, just behind the fog. I understand that you are there right now. And I want to let you know that I understand that something happened. You were given this anesthetic, and you may think that this is how the world is or what you are. And I'm so sorry that you had to go through that. Even though we were all doing our best, I can only guess that you couldn't feel me, and that might have been really scary. You may have even thought I wasn't okay, or that I was dead or you were. I want to let you know that I'm okay and I'm so sorry that happened to you. I promise I won't let that happen again, and I can feel you are here too. I'm so sorry that at that time I didn't know this was happening to you.*

If you start describing what you see — "I see that you are tense or angry" or "I see that you're floppy or sleeping or going away with your attention, or foggy behind your eyes" — you have a chance to deeply connect at the place of the baby's most troubling wound. By slowly making your way through an imagining of what it might have been like in a particular situation, you will gradually touch on the baby's honest responses, your own empathy, and the sincere grief shared by both of you for the situation. By adding statements that show empathy, regret, and differentiation (that is, making it clear that what happened is separate from the baby), you can truly be a healing resource for a child. End by thanking the baby for coming to you, make it clear that "I'm always here, and I'm so sorry it happened," promise to never let this happen again, and remind the baby that you are so glad he or she is here, and that even though a cesarean might have been the best decision at that time, you know he or she was hurt.

Because babies delivered by cesarean are born in a way not of their choosing, and because they will have missed the much-needed rhythmic pressure of the last stages of birth, they will usually want more physical contact and containment than other babies. The best thing you can do is agree to their needs, even if other babies seem to be acting more "independently." Babies know what they need, and they know their natural pace.

Rushing them or shaming them for wanting to be close will harm their confidence and delay their independence, potentially for a lifetime. It may even teach them to give up on asking for contact and support.

If you are the baby who is revisiting feelings from many years ago, you can treat yourself in the same ways I've described above, as though you are talking to your own baby, but the baby is you! You may still need to finish your own birth, and finding a skilled practitioner and the appropriate environment to help you do that will be life changing.

Healing for Toddlers

If the effects of a cesarean birth are left unaddressed, toddlers often try to regain their lost choice by becoming very assertive about what they will or won't eat, what they will or won't wear, and how and when they enter and exit rooms, cars, and other locations. As with the other types of birth interventions discussed earlier, these are examples of children attempting to regain their choice. A key to their healing is avoiding entering into power struggles with them. Congratulate them and offer empathy, saying something like, "*You didn't have the choice back then, but you are choosing now.*" Celebrate their choice!

This effort to regain control is over and above the toddler's common and necessary stage of saying "no" to everything. You must achieve a fine balance when caring for a child who says, "I won't eat that," or who won't let himself poop, or won't leave a room. How do you honour the child's need to regain choice, while still fulfilling your responsibility to care for and protect the child?

Congratulating children and toddlers for asserting their choice and showing what they want, and letting them know how excited that makes you, at least puts you on their side. Letting them see how sad you are that they ever lost their choice in the first place is also very powerful. As soon as children understand that someone else knows how hard it was for them or how scary or frustrating or life-and-death it was, as soon as someone else gets it, they don't have to keep on telling the story by resisting the things that are happening to them. If children put themselves in a situation that exceeds your sense of what's safe or doable, you can tell them:

I see you are making a choice. Yay! That is fantastic! And I'm so sorry you had that taken from you before. I was there, I know what happened. It was a big deal, and I get that now. (You can add more sentences that come from your heart.) And, it's my job to take care of you, so I'm bringing you with me, or inviting you to do (x) with me.

Even if children fight and scream after you've said these validating things, their need to protect themselves will decrease as they see that you are willing to do whatever it takes to protect them.

Some practitioners I know teach parents how to play protection games with their children. In these games, a stuffed animal with mean intentions is dramatized as coming for the child. The parents either bring another stuffed animal to protect the child from the mal-intending toy, or stand in themselves to show the child they are strong enough to protect her. For a parent who was at a birth and felt helpless, it can be very healing to reclaim the position as the protector!

The Ideal Cesarean Birth

Robert Oliver, an obstetrician, spent the bulk of his career administering birth interventions according to conventional medical wisdom. Thirty-five years into his practice, he had an epiphany. He summarized his revelations in an article he wrote called "The Ideal Cesarean Birth."

> *For the first time I looked at my work with pregnant women and realized that although I was getting great medical results I was getting terrible results for the woman with regard to her needs and self-esteem; and, I was unconscious of the baby and of the effects of standard care on this new person.*
>
> *I hated these things. I hated the thought that all my good intentions were wrong. I hated knowing I had not been giving appropriately to what should be vital in the transformative event of birth — the woman transformed into mother and the conceptus into a new human being. I hated knowing the shortcuts I took during long labour — operative delivery by forceps and cesarean section just to get on with it; the inductions of labour for my own convenience not for the safety and integrity of the woman; the application of technique and technology to make my job safer from lawsuit and peer criticism and*

to meet demands of hospital policy. I remember and recognize the anger I felt at women who wanted natural childbirth, home delivery and non-intervention. I am ashamed, and I am also satisfied that whereas I was once stupid but medically sound, I am now awake and profoundly aware that I know nothing about the experience of gestation, birthing, and the transformative experience of becoming a mother. I can only view it, this process a woman passes into, from the outside as a father, a man, and a professional male in obstetrics.[35]

Farther along in his article, Dr. Oliver describes how he learned that it was essential for the entire surgical team to be intentional with their emotions and send love to the baby and mother prior to even administering anesthetic.[36] He recommended talking to the baby before any changes in the mother's body, to say, "These hands that are coming in are here to help and love you."[37] He goes on to describe how he uses his hands to transform the surgical wound into a birth canal and lets the baby continue to contract and push through his hands. He waits until the umbilical cord stops pulsing before clamping it from the placenta. He helps the mother, the father or partner, and the birthing team stay connected to the baby throughout the procedure. The courage Dr. Oliver reveals in his honest telling of the transformation he went through shows us that it is indeed possible to incorporate medical procedures into conscious, gentle birth. There is a way to save lives and prevent harm using emergency measures while applying loving intentions.

CASE STUDY: *Cara, Peter and Lily*

Cara's labour started slowly. She was in steady contractions for three days and was exhausted. Although Cara was a strong, mature woman, the nurses and midwives were keeping a close watch on her fluid levels and on her baby's heart rate. At some point near the end of the third day, the obstetrician suggested they might need to do a cesarean to avoid risking the baby's health. Cara was reluctant to have a cesarean. She had had a healthy pregnancy, natural birth was in line with her values, and she had worked hard over the past few days to attain that. Although she was exhausted, she was mentally and physically prepared to continue with the labour.

Cara and her husband, Peter, were no strangers to trusting their baby's intelligence. They had conceived their baby with full awareness that her soul was coming to join them. At the time of her conception, which was achieved with the assistance of technology, they had planned and carried out a ceremony, and they had continued communicating with the baby over the months she was growing in Cara's womb. Although Cara and Peter shared their belief in the value of unmedicated vaginal birth, they also knew that such a long labour was surely hard on their baby, so they remained open-minded while Cara communicated with the baby. "Okay, little one, if you need us to come in there and get you, you let me know."

Cara says the answer came right away. Within seconds, her baby's heart rate dropped. It was at that moment that Cara made the unequivocal decision to have a cesarean. She knew her baby was communicating with her.

Cara, Peter, and the hospital team delivered Lily by cesarean fifteen minutes later. Lily's head had been wedged in Cara's uterus and was misshapen from the days of pressure. Cara and Peter immediately began to speak with Lily, knowing she could understand them. They let her know that their long birth must have hurt and must have been scary, and they let her know they were going to do everything necessary to help her work out any lasting effects the particular challenges of her birth had left her with.

Years later, Lily has grown into a girl who trusts herself and knows her desires. The edges on her skull have smoothed so they are barely noticeable to the touch, and the communicative relationship she forged with her parents during her gestation and birth continues between them today.

CASE STUDY: *Karen, John and Joshua*

Karen phoned to say she'd like me to meet with her and her family. Their elder son, Joshua, then three and a half, was often overwhelmed or afraid, and would say upsetting things to his parents or to other children he was playing with. Karen suspected his challenges had something to do with his birth.

Karen told me that when he was playing with other children, Joshua would go through several seconds of crying. Then he would become angry, bury his head in Karen's shoulder, and say, "I want to cut their heads off. I want to destroy them. I want them to go!"

It's easy to appreciate Karen and John's concerns. Most parents are keenly aware of their desire to raise children who are cooperative and non-violent.

When I asked Karen and John about Joshua's birth, they described a long labour, which included an airlift to a hospital as the family lived in a remote location. Karen received an epidural, and Joshua was eventually born by cesarean. When a doctor explained the challenges they had faced during his birth, he told Karen that Joshua's "head was too big."

During our first session, I encouraged Karen and John to try looking at Joshua's responses as memories being awoken. What I meant was that present circumstances, either at home or while playing with other children, somehow reminded Joshua of his birth. His choice of words — "I want to cut their heads off" — seemed to me an accurate way to describe what it's like when one's head is being pulled on during a cesarean. Aside from a small handful of babies who were born by elective cesarean under intentional and loving circumstances, every baby I've treated who was born by cesarean has leftover face, head, neck, and/or shoulder injuries from the events. And even though a baby's tissues do their best to heal after the initial injury, pain and fears persist because the baby, and likely the mother, has not yet been able to work through the deeper tissue injuries and emotional grief.

Joshua was telling us his story in several ways. For example, when I asked him, "What was it like for you?" he took his stuffed toy rabbit and pushed the rabbit's ears down. When I responded, "Oh, that's what it was like for you? Oh, that must have hurt," he either crawled into his father's lap and curled up in the fetal position or crawled inside a fort of pillows he had assembled.

Over several sessions together, we encouraged Joshua to find his way out of his chosen tucked-in places by letting him push off us using his feet and his low back. Sometimes, during his exits, he would get stalled, almost stuck. Especially during those times, we would acknowledge him for showing us what it was like for him, and we would offer our empathy and remorse for how frustrated and scared he felt when he was stuck.

When I asked Joshua where it hurt, he would show me by using toys to point to his right eye and nose. Again, we'd offer words of empathy and remorse.

Never did I consider that Joshua was growing into a violent or mal-intending young boy. Although violence is within the range of human qualities, children are not likely to come up with such graphic and specific fears unless they have witnessed something similar. If parents are loving and available, and still their child is saying things that sound violent or hateful, it's important to look at the circumstances of the child's birth. Babies do know what's happening to them, they do have feelings about what's happening, and, like Joshua, they do remember them. When they are not able to understand where their irritation, fear, anger, or sadness is coming from, children revert to words and actions like Joshua did. They want us to understand and will tell us the best way they know how.

Over several sessions, Joshua freed himself from his fort of pillows or from his father's lap in various, creative ways, sometimes with our help, and sometimes on his own. Each time he moved out of his seemingly tightly bound position, he had a smile, as though to say, "Look what I've done!"

After our last session I happened to run into Joshua's grandmother, who lived a few minutes' walk from the family's house. She said to me, "Mia, I have to thank you. Although I know Joshua has always loved me and felt close to me, he's never said my name, 'Gramma.' It's pained me, but I've tried to be patient. Today, after your session, I walked in the house and he welcomed me with 'Gramma!' I'm so grateful to you." Joshua's grandmother had tears in her eyes. I could see how Joshua's suffering had prevented him from connecting with her. Now that he was freed to feel more himself, he could better acknowledge those around him, and he had access to words that described what he knew on the inside.

CASE STUDY: *Sylvie and Terrence*

Sylvie reached out to say she wanted support for herself and her son, Terrence, after their birth. She had been working at her recovery for several years, as Terrence was already four years old.

The birth had included a hospital transfer from a remote location after what she had hoped would be a natural home birth. Once in the hospital, Sylvie was given nitrous oxide (laughing gas), and Terrence was eventually delivered with the use of forceps and a C-section. Sylvie explained that a large part of the trauma of her birth had to do with miscommunication and lack of continuity of care between those who were assisting her birth at home and those who assisted her in the hospital. For a birthing mother, stability, safety, tenderness, and continuity of care are essential if her body is to open and birth her child.

Terrence was separated from Sylvie for a time after he was born. Doctors cleaned Terrence's mouth and nose with suction somewhere far away from Sylvie, and once she was wheeled out of surgery into the recovery room, Terrence, now held by his father, was taken elsewhere so he could be cleaned and heel pricked.

Thankfully, Terrence did nurse when he was finally brought back to Sylvie.

Sylvie, her partner, and Terrence went home from the hospital. Ten days later, Sylvie's incision wound ruptured, and an enormous amount of pus burst out. She was immediately flown back to the hospital for emergency surgery.

Four and a half years later, when I met Terrence for the first time, Sylvie explained to me that he had been "holding his poop in" since he began taking solid food at eighteen months. More recently, he began pinching her face quite hard and saying, "I'm going to kill you, kill Daddy, and I'm going to kill myself!"

Because I don't consider children to be inherently violent or ill-meaning, I suspected Terrence was describing his own experience. When mothers are anesthetized and cannot feel their babies, babies believe their mothers, their world, and therefore they themselves are going to die. During his birth, Terrence must have felt like his mom or his father was killed, and that he had been killed, perhaps as a consequence of their deaths.

We played with Terrence, encouraging him to show us what it was like for him to be born, or what it felt like to be him. He said, "An egg gets turned on and becomes a baby and it grows until it has to come out." Then he went on to say, "The blood wanted to stay in the heart and didn't want to come out." He would also repeat, "I just want to stay on Momma's belly" and "I want to go back inside with Mama."

I suspected what he meant was that he hadn't finished lingering in stages of development while in his mother's womb, and that he certainly would have preferred to birth the way he wanted to do it. Since he was unable to do that, he "wanted back in."

When we played with him, using our hands to support his body so he could show us what he wanted to do, he would repeatedly lie on his stomach and push his way along the floor and into Sylvie's arms. To me, this looked like he was getting a chance to do the vaginal birth all mammals are born to do. This encouraged me, because if babies, children, or even adults get a chance to complete their birth, not in an idea or as a performance, but in a deep way arising from instincts inside their bodies, as Terrence was doing, they can move on in their development, feel more confident and safe in the world, and heal their bodies from pain and misalignment.

Sylvie told me that throughout his early years, Terrence was very resistant to having water in his face. During a later session, Terrence said, "I'll spray dirty poopy water in your mouth." This made me think he may have remembered being suctioned and painfully separated from his mother. We offered him compassion and regret that this happened to him. Sylvie and her partner discovered a few weeks later that Terrence was no longer afraid to put his head under the shower spray!

Sylvie related another profound aspect of their story, not to be underestimated, when she told me how, as she was giving birth to Terrence in the hospital, she was wearing a necklace that signalled she was part of an unconventional spiritual practice. As attuned as she was, and despite the distraction from the chaos of giving birth and making the decision to have a C-section, Sylvie was sure she had perceived moral or religious judgment coming from her doctor while he was performing her surgery and sewing her up.

When I did a session with Sylvie on her own (which is often important for mothers to do after birth), I worked on the area where her cesarean scar was. It was then that she had a deep insight, followed by a release of grief at how the doctor's judgment had influenced her tissues. Her sense was that her wound had not healed and had become dangerously infected because of her lack of trust in him, requiring her to return to the hospital for another emergency surgery.

The Fourth Stage of Labour

According to French obstetrician Michel Odent, labour is complete when the placenta is delivered.[38] Ray Castellino and Mary Jackson, leaders in pre- and perinatal therapy, believe that birth extends beyond the moment a baby is born, and is over once the child first sucks and swallows colostrum (the densely nutritious liquid that precedes breast milk for four days).[39] What is significant about the fourth stage of labour?

Self-attachment or Attachment Sequencing, described in Chapter 3, is the series of natural gestures every mammal makes right after birth, which includes finding the way to the breast. Humans are no different. People are so accustomed to babies being swaddled and lifted to the breast after birth and at home that they are shocked to discover birth actually includes a long and patient journey to the nipple. This delicate and extremely significant event may last twenty minutes or it may go on as long as an hour.

After a baby is born, he spends the first fifteen or twenty minutes just getting used to breathing on his own. He needs about that long to start clearing his lungs. This means there's no need to rush to nurse; it's okay to put a baby on his mother's stomach and just let him spend time there. This allows him to adjust and build potency in his nervous system to make the next journey.

The contractions that he and his mother make during labour are now translating into impulses that will help him wriggle and begin the journey toward his mother's breast. Ideally, mother and baby should have skin-to-skin contact with nothing obstructing the baby's route. The key chemical, oxytocin, will sustain babies and mothers if they can feel each other's skin. The mother will want to be warm and relaxed. It is best not to cut the cord until the placenta is delivered and the umbilical cord stops pulsing.[40] Everyone in the room might consider resisting the urge to "do things" at this time. Keep the lights low, slow down, talk quietly or not at all, and use light touch and gentle words to encourage the baby to find his way.

Some babies need more time to reach the breast. They may be processing what happened during the birth or earlier in their development. They may pause or even appear stuck on their way to the breast. This gives them a chance to work out what went on between them and their mothers just before birth, while they were in the womb. Of course, this pause may have echoes of what's in the Family Field as well. Babies will slow down and make noises. Through these noises and their body movements, babies are, for the first time in the outside world, beginning to tell their story. Giving babies support at their feet can help if some places are a little more "stuck" than others.

Some babies do not latch the first time if sections of labour were challenging or traumatic for their systems. These babies may be able to suckle after they have had a chance to tell their story enough times. If babies appear to lack sufficient strength or potency to travel and self-attach, there are gentle and encouraging ways to stimulate them. Roughly rubbing their bodies, or moving them rapidly, will only overwhelm them further.

In cases where self-attachment is missed, like during a necessary life-saving medical intervention in which the mother and baby must be separated, Attachment Sequencing can be played like a game after the baby is born. Allowing time every day to self-attach gives babies the reward and encouragement of "finding their way" and connecting with love and support. The result is that as they grow up, babies will bring all their feelings to their parents. A mother can even try letting her baby find his way to her breast from higher up on her chest while holding him. Her baby will slowly creep down toward his breast of choice if allowed to put his face and body on his mother.

Self-attachment has been known to happen after a cesarean, and even hours after birth if babies have been separated from their mothers. Some people have experienced their first self-attachment sequence in adulthood while in a healing milieu. It is never too late to experience moments of bonding.

Separation

Babies may have imprints from separation when they have been taken away from their mother after birth. They could be taken away for washing, suctioning, drops, heal pricks, or testing, or because their mother is unavailable due to medical emergency or to receive stitches for an episiotomy. Premature babies are taken from their mother and father to the neonatal intensive care unit (NICU). Some NICUs have adopted systems to keep parents in close contact with their babies, while others have not.[41] Babies may be separated for minutes — which seem like lifetimes to them and their mothers — or they may be separated for months (depending on how the NICU functions).

Because babies need to bond with someone or something, and because brain development and adaptation to the world depend on bonding, whoever or whatever is there at and after birth will become a reference point for their world. This works well when love, comfort, and connection are present. A baby, later a child, will seek similar feelings throughout life. If pain or isolation are present, and are left untreated, those feelings will form a norm and will be sought throughout life. Many women have told me "My partner seems to be able to soothe my baby better than me" and then revealed that they were unfortunately separated from their baby due to a medical emergency. Sadly, babies who initially spend more time with machines, lights, and incubators than their parents will become closer to machines than to people. They must come into relationship if they are to survive, and they will do so with anything. Babies that have been separated can get reminded of the pain of the separation when they are given an opportunity to be close with their mothers.

Both babies and mothers require lots of compassion for being separated.

Healing for Mothers

Long after birth is over, even years later, mothers report that being separated from their baby still affects them. They wish they could go back to that time and do things differently, over and above any other intervention. This is why it is important for mothers to be given time to have their story heard, with lots of compassion and regret offered to them, even if it is years later. Only after they have received support for what they went through will they have enough compassion to truly hear the hurt in their baby or child.

A unique challenge that arises after all birth interventions is that mothers and babies think they are not close. They think their relationship lacks a bond. Very often it is the intervention that got between them and is still lodged there. Separation after birth is the most dramatic block to being close. If babies and mothers are anesthetized, that block to their closeness sits even more deeply in their cellular experiences. The mother, and then the mother and baby, can and must work through those layers if their bond is to feel strong and real to them both.

Healing for Babies

To heal separation, parents need to address all the details, known and guessed at, that came into play between birth and the time the baby was reunited with her mother. Babies can feel betrayed or shocked; they may fear that their mother is dead and therefore they're going to die or should be dead; and there are many other possible fears and experiences. Talking to babies about what happened to them is key. If they are fascinated by machines, lights, and even strangers (if they bonded with the nurses, for example), it is important that you acknowledge this as something they did to get by while separated from you. If you encourage them to show you how the early hours or weeks of their life shaped them, you indicate how much you respect their desire to live and let them know that you are not trying to take that away from them.

Babies who were separated at birth and now seem to prefer things other than their mother or father have done a brilliant thing in that they chose life! They will eventually want to return to human contact, but for now that preference is buried under the grief of being separated, which is buried under their preference for other things. The goal is not to take away their preferences, but to non-forcefully become available by slowly telling them their story with compassion, regret, and reminders that they are not the lights, the sounds, or the strangers; that you are here and available; and that they can come to you at their own pace.

Initially, babies may avert their gaze or not want to be near their parents. The loss for babies is so overwhelming that they may not be able to withstand the grief that rises in them when they are close to their mother's body. What may look like rejection of their mother is in fact a strong cry to have what happened to them made known. A reparative gesture for babies who have been separated is to let them know what's happening before it happens — for example, "I'm changing you now" or "I'm passing you to so-and-so now" or "I'm giving you my breast now." Anything that can telegraph what's happening before it happens will help reduce their need to protect themselves and will rebuild trust.

Babies who had meconium (their first poop, which can be expelled while they are still in the womb and then inhaled) or fluids removed from their nose or mouth by suction right after birth typically remember the procedure as incredibly invasive and scary, and probably painful. When some babies go to nurse, they can be reminded of the sudden shock of suction in their mouth or nose, and they pull away from the breast because of it. Babies' feet can be sensitive because of heel pricks, their eyes can be sensitive because of drops they were given. There are all sorts of practices in and even out of hospitals that can be extraneous and startling, as well as surprising and traumatizing to babies. When parents open their curiosity and remind themselves that any adverse responses are usually the result of memories being awakened, they are better equipped to support their babies.

Talk to your baby, saying things like *"I'm so sorry that happened to you, I see what you're showing me"* or

> *I don't understand what happened, but I'm trying to imagine and I'd really like to know. Whatever it is, I'm so sorry that it happened. I really wanted to be with you and protect you and be close to you and know you and love you. And I want to let you know that the separation, when you were with that machine and were away from me, or that pressure in your nose and mouth when you were being suctioned, that's not who you are. These are the things that happened to you.*

These same words can apply if your child is older or if it was you who was separated from your mother and father after birth. With children, watch for expressions of anger or grief after you talk to them. Their response may delay for days or even weeks, but there will be one. If you are the child, keep speaking to yourself. Initially it may feel staged or contrived. Eventually, real feelings will surface. When they do, love yourself as the "good parent" would. Show yourself compassion and regret for what happened. The consequences of separation will lessen in intensity with sustained, consistent compassion, no matter your child's or your age.

NICU and Surgery

The neonatal intensive care unit (NICU) is a specialized area of the hospital that cares for babies who are born before they are fully grown, so cannot live on their own outside the womb, or are born with health complications requiring various forms of life support or close monitoring. As mentioned earlier, stays in the NICU can last for minutes, days, or as long as weeks and months, depending on the baby's health challenges.

The NICU is one of the most caring and attuned areas of the hospital, where, thanks to the intelligent use of technology; highly trained staff, nurses, and doctors; and an enormous amount of compassion, lives continue when they otherwise wouldn't.

Most NICUs attempt to keep parents as close to their babies as possible, even when babies must spend time in an *isolette*, or incubator. In some cases, however, parents may not want to see their babies. This could occur when parents are unable to contend with the shock they've already experienced and are not equipped to deal with the possible death of their baby or the life with a high-needs infant that awaits them. There is a range of responses in the NICU.

Parents whose children are in the NICU go through enormous stress for the reasons mentioned in the previous paragraph, but also because of the amount of time spent away from home, daily life, and possibly other children. They require support in the form of friendship, counselling, and bodywork, if only to discharge the stress.

Babies in the NICU, because of their challenges, often receive better care than babies who are born at term. Imprints from premature birth should be expected, however, even though parents are unusually focused on their love and gratitude for this child's life.

Some of the health challenges babies in the NICU have are similar to those associated with other birth imprints we've discussed. In addition, they will have digestive challenges, respiratory challenges, and, depending on their age, very sensitive skin, hyper-sensitive hearing, and acute response to attention and other people's desires. While all babies are very sensitive to signals from around them, NICU babies have fewer resources with which to integrate the stimulus coming from around and within them. While they often look docile, their internal world likely feels overwhelming, unprotected, and painful. They may also be fully aware of their importance to others, as many people are caring for them.

Many NICU babies will be very particular about who they get emotionally close to as babies, and later as children and adults. They may find it hard to bond in a love relationship or to expose themselves emotionally because of how big feelings were and still are for them. Because they were separated for so long, even if they were able to spend some time with their parents and nurses, they will have bonded with the incubator walls, the catheters, the blood pressure cuffs, and the sound of the machines around them. And yet, because they were so dearly cared for by the NICU nurses, and like all babies, were hungry for connection, they will have their own unique bonding dynamics later in life.

It is essential that parents use the same language and sensitivity with them as with other babies, offering compassion and remorse, as well as speaking to what they see in NICU babies to help differentiate their sensitivities, making it clear that these feelings come from their experiences and are not their identity.

Consulting the Family Field is an important step of recovery after coming home and adjusting from being in the NICU. As mentioned in Chapter 2, historical events can influence how birth plays out. For example, events as recent as the mother facing high demands before or during pregnancy related to work or unforeseen circumstances like an illness or death in her family. It's not uncommon for birth to come early when a mother is under-resourced. Babies can be in NICUs for reasons other than prematurity, like challenges with breathing or digesting. All physiological symptoms present at birth have roots in the embryonic period or in earlier history before the child was conceived. Some of the reasons may remain a mystery, but through quiet and curious reflection, the support of a pre-birth and birth-trained therapist, and exploration of your Family Field, you may get glimpses of understanding.

NICU experiences are shocking for parents as well as meaningful. The consequences of the stress build up over months and are sometimes not addressed until long after the baby's hospital stay. The intense emotions and careful care during the stay can make for a strong bond throughout life. Osteopathy, craniosacral therapy, counselling, and the compassion of community will help parents release the stress they carried from that time and help them integrate what they learned and carry it forward into their daily life and parenting.

As mentioned, all birth interventions can be transformed into positive experiences by using the awareness and tools offered in this section. The global medical community is coming to see that birth needs to be protected and that there are lasting consequences when the natural process is interrupted. This means we may see a drop in birth interventions over the next several decades. Because the change will be slow, we must continue to look at how we can integrate the results of interventions while they are still in such abundance.

Adult Recovery

Birth imprints shape adult behavior just like prebirth ones. The effects are myriad, so they cannot be predicted, and yet distinct aspects of adult life are consistently altered: For example, physical posture; physical sensitivity; intuitive and emotional sensitivity; quality of touch; relationship to time and timing; capacity for intimacy; rhythm of intimacy; mental clarity; capacity to be present; learning; learning retention; sense of safety and trust; capacity for pleasure; capacity for joy; and capacity for compassion.

How can you examine whether your birth still affects you? One way is to work backwards. Whether your birth was troublesome or wonderful, it left a trail. The trail begins in your present-day life. Begin your inquiry by examining any aspect of the present. For example, how do you engage with projects or tasks? Do you favour the beginning, middle, or end? During which stage do you get bogged down? Which stage moves smoothly, and when in the timeline do you tend to lose interest, enjoyment, or stop working all together? Follow these clues back to your birth. It's likely they map fairly closely onto how your birth started, progressed, and completed. What if you discover that you're a great starter, but a terrible finisher? How do you transform that? One option is to give yourself compassion when you find yourself losing contact with the project or task. Assume you're having a memory, even if you don't know what it is. Imagine yourself as a good mother or father, lovingly holding the baby you once were, until the aversive or even 'cut-off' sensations subside. You might find after doing this that it's easier to pick the thread up again and continue what you were working on. Sometime you'll even have a spontaneous memory in the form of grief or anger come up while you're nurturing your young self. Acknowledge your young self for providing you with this memory, for having the courage to tell you the truth.

Birthdays are opportune times to detect birth imprints. Some people get excited in anticipation of their approaching birthday, but come the day, they feel alone and insecure. Some feel trepidation leading up to the day, but flourish when it finally arrives. Perhaps someone was excitedly anticipating your arrival before or on the day you were born! You might have had a combination of experiences, such as in the case where you might have been excited to be born, but you got the impression others weren't because you got injured by birth imprints or were separated from your mother. Feel into it. You'll discover the nuances pertaining to your unique history. If you encounter uncomfortable feelings, give empathy to the young one who is telling you about them. Thank your young one, and let her know you are available if there is more to learn.

Your body is able to take you on a tour of your birth. If you were born with forceps, vacuum extraction, or forceps during cesarean, you might still have pain in your head, neck, upper back, or in your lower back and hips. Although birth is naturally full of force, the force is spread out evenly over your whole body, and is naturally mitigated with the help of endogenous endorphins. Sometimes up to seventy pounds of pressure are used with forceps. That's a lot of force applied to a very small and sensitive area. Tissues around the brain, in your neck, upper back, and torso will take that force so your brain doesn't have to bear the brunt. Pain that seems to come out of nowhere, and is only temporarily subdued by stretching muscles, can often arise from underlying connective tissue, organs, and ligaments injured at birth.

Vacuum extractions also pull on the fine membranes around the brain, which will automatically traction the connective tissue throughout the spinal cord, affecting multiple areas around your body, particularly the base of your skull, your palate, your diaphragm and your pelvic floor. These physical traumas and others involving physical strain can be helped by osteopaths and craniosacral therapists trained in pre and perinatal dynamics. However the trauma manifests, giving your young self empathy whenever your present life reminds you of the circumstances of your birth is critical to healing.

It's possible to recall the effects of anesthetics in your present day life. Depending on the nature of the chemicals used to anesthetize your mother, the duration they were used for, and the dose, along with how much you were held and connected with after birth will shape the degree to which they've lingered with you. Common adult leftovers from anesthetics are a 'haze', 'fog', or 'cloudiness' that sits like a drape or a barrier between you and others, or you and the world. Some people feel like they are 'outside of life' while others are 'in it'. This barrier can increase when we're called to be emotionally or physically intimate with another. It can arise when someone near you makes a bid for your care or compassion. Having received anesthetics (through your mother) in the form of epidural, sedatives, general anesthetic, opioids, or other dissociative drugs during birth could make you feel 'cold', 'floaty', 'blank', 'far away', 'fuzzy', or 'sleepy', even though your personality is warm, affectionate, energetic, and enthusiastic. Anesthetics might also have been used for a procedure or surgery after you were born. This too could contribute to a feeling of separateness from others and the world.

Try dissolving the effect of anesthetics by asking to connect with a deeper presence within you that lives beneath the foggy overlay. Say to yourself, "this is who I am", and concentrate on a layer of your presence that doesn't feel foggy, especially when you feel the memory coming on. Human capacity for intimacy has suffered for generations because of anesthetics given to mothers at birth. These chemicals also shape societal norms by convincing mothers that they should not hold their children or respond to their cries. Mothers simply cannot arouse themselves if anesthetized. If anesthetic was introduced during the birth, mothers are less likely to respond to their children, even for several hours after birth. Without this awareness, the habit imprints their bond, and could later influence how you bond. With steady practice, however, this habit can lessen and even dissolve.

Timing is a facet of life that is heavily imprinted by birth. If your birth was intervened upon, this might possibly be the first time you encountered 'time out of Nature'. People whose births were sped up, prolonged, or rushed through induction, augmentation, epidural, forceps, vacuum, and cesarean have had their natural timing taken from them. Just like the babies and children you read about earlier, when something intrinsic like sovereign timing has been violated, the urge to right it never ends. For this reason you might feel the need to arrive early or feel trepidation at being late. This is often a memory of being rushed during birth, of having to 'get there before you get there'. Chronic lateness might be related to birth memories. If you were rushed, you might be reclaiming the right to your own timing, and prefer to delay if you sense any attempt at tyranny over your own sovereign rhythms. Once at events you might want to stay on the periphery, need to be in the middle, or possibly, never want to arrive at all. Detect your habit, and become curious about it. Offer yourself empathy if strong feelings come up about it. Nurture yourself as a good mother or father until the feeling subsides. Remind yourself you have now have choice when originally you didn't. It is a tragedy that your sovereignty, through the manipulation of time, was taken from you at the beginning. Someone needed to have acknowledged and shown regret about this right away. If they didn't, it's understandable that you would still have feelings about it. It's likely that you are still trying to reclaim your choice today.

One way to work with your discomfort with time, or your wish to reclaim it back, is to become aware of it. Just like with chemical imprints, you have an authentic self that lives beneath the manipulated level of timing in your tissues. Connect with it; announce to yourself that this is your sovereign being. Make a choice from this deeper place. It's a freeing act. Give yourself permission to only do what you really want to do, and you will heal much of the coercion that was placed on you before you could fight for your rights to your own timing. If you fear that doing only what you want to do might ruin your relationships, then let those you love know that you're experimenting with healing your birth, and that you'd like their understanding while you do it.

Your present day habits, be they avoiding contact, dialing back your presence, arriving late, diving into the center of the conversation of the party, even when it's not warranted, or staying on the outside, are always an expression of your desire for freedom. You are saying, 'never again will I be trapped and tortured the way I was when I was too young and powerless to respond and fight. Good for you! You might have noticed that other people don't always like the way you reclaim your freedom. It's okay to consider their feedback. Perhaps you've been reclaiming lost power in the best way you've known up until now. With this new awareness, you can make a more informed choice about how you'd like to reinstate power that was taken from you.

Birth recovery provides you with options. Are you are really trapped in the present, or is the present reminding you of the past? Could you arrive on time without too much anxiety for being late? Could you show up to the event, the conversation, or the lovemaking and see if by taking a short break, you can quell the discomfort that is making you want to leave or interrupt? Can you trust that by asking for more of what you want, you'll feel less afraid and more connected? Trust your preferences. Grant yourself freedom– always. It could be that where you are or whom you're with is not a fit. It could be that the other person is such a fit that they call you to heal everything that stands in the way of your communion. Experiment.

Delving into imprinted birth memories is not for the faint of heart. Looking at them takes courage, the willingness to sit with heart-breaking feelings, and the capacity to be present to the young baby in you. If our society can learn to restore trust, safety, and connection to our youngest selves, we open the gateway for future generations to enjoy greater well-being. We also open the gateway to having a better exit in that our deaths stand to become the sacred threshold we wished our births had been.

CHAPTER 6

When Babies Don't Survive

As mentioned earlier, babies are the ones to initiate birth. Some arrive earlier than planned but can be kept alive in an NICU. Other babies will have a very premature birth — arriving so early that they cannot be kept alive by technology. We call that family's experience a *miscarriage* or, if it occurs in the sixty days after conception, *early pregnancy loss*. Some babies are never born, and their bodies are discovered on x-ray; some babies have vanished altogether by way of what can only be called the Great Mystery.

All these babies are babies. All of them have a life, if only for a short time. All of their parents have become parents, if only for a short time.

Miscarriage

Without doubt, miscarriage is society's most hidden kind of birth. For women and their families, miscarriage is incredibly painful and surprisingly common. One in four women will experience a miscarriage or stillbirth in their lifetimes. This means that there are a lot of children who have never been acknowledged in the Family Fields. Even if miscarriage happens when a woman or her family are reluctant to have their child, the long-lasting effects can be deep.

Indigenous wisdom holds that souls are present early in pregnancy, as early as in the first few weeks. I have worked with people who recall being sentient even before they were conceived. For this reason, it is important for families to acknowledge that a child did in fact come to them, even if the child did not stay past two, six, eight, twelve, or even twenty weeks.

After a miscarriage, a woman will experience a profound hormonal flux, which can make her feel depressed and despairing, and may even cause unexplainable weight gain and acne. Depending on how much blood is lost (usually proportional to the age of her embryo or fetus at the time of death), she may emerge from the birth with low iron or anemia. In this case, she will be exhausted, sad, and unable to satisfy her hunger or quell her grief.

Healing from Miscarriage

It's important that a mother be cared for by others after a miscarriage. It's also important to tend to the father. Ideally, a woman must be kept physically warm. This keeps her body relaxed by preventing an increase in stress hormones. Give a woman light food to eat. Soups and broths help her body concentrate on restoring strength. Bone broths, Indian dhals (lentil soups), and vegetable soups are best in the first week, and bone broths afterwards will help restore her iron.

Even if she doesn't want to rest, she must. A miscarriage that occurs after eight weeks will typically take more from her than one at four weeks, but in either case her body will still be in shock, and she shouldn't be challenged by exertion like carrying more than a pound or two, excessive socializing, too much planning, or anything that takes her away from being able to feel her feelings. She should be encouraged to put her feet up a couple of times a day. If there is a naturopath in your area, she will benefit from receiving injections of folic acid and other micronutrients a couple of times a week for at least two weeks. Proper dietary and hormonal support can mitigate future miscarriages, and these factors are worth investigating. If repeated miscarriage occurs, especially late in the first trimester, it can be an indication of adrenal fatigue or other hormonal imbalances. Consulting a naturopath is a good idea.

When a child miscarries, a woman often feels she's done something wrong or that there is something intrinsically wrong with her. Fathers may also want to take on this misplaced responsibility. It is true that the age of eggs and sperms, the presence of chemicals in parents' bodies, and many other physical factors can play a role in miscarriage, but even after tangible

health factors are accounted for, there are still many unexplained miscarriages. However, for both parents, trying to take full responsibility has more
to do with their inability to fully accept that this baby will never grow and
be born. This is a painful reality, and the suffering it causes often brings
up other, older, ungrieved suffering as well. The parents have no control
over what has happened and must be supported to grieve both their child
and their powerlessness in the face of the unknown.

Men need to be supported by their fellow men, especially elder men, who
have seen many of life's challenges and can lend their presence, easing the
burden a man feels about the challenges he and his partner are having.
Women should be supported by other women. A woman who has been
through a miscarriage may be of even greater solace than women who,
though they are loving and compassionate, cannot fully relate.

Bearing the grief and the powerlessness is a capacity both the mother
and father must develop. It is grown by letting their loss be known, by
having a ceremony with friends and family where they can share their grief,
by resisting moving on too quickly and looking to conceive immediately.
The chance to try again can bring solace, but should not replace the space
this child who never arrived occupies. Although women who miscarry are
often eager to conceive again very soon afterwards, taking the time to grieve
and restore offers a happier and healthier pregnancy later, and lessens
mothers' fears that they may lose another child.

When families conceive another child, and that child stays on to be
born, it is important to let the new child know there was once (or however
many times you've miscarried) another one there, so this new child does
not come to resonate with the death that happened, thinking it happened
to him or her. The "haunted womb" is a term used in pre- and perinatal
psychology to describe the "echo" left by an unborn miscarried child that
has never been grieved.

Ceremony

Consider planning and carrying out a ritual or ceremony to honour the
very young life that has died. I have spoken to many women who were
not told to do this or never thought of doing it, and even decades later
they have told me that they were never able to fully honour the child or
children they miscarried. One woman even shared with me that for some

reason she "thinks of the child who miscarried almost more than [her] other children."

Indigenous customs will have the mother and her partner create a place to honour their child. Go to the woods, or somewhere in nature outside of your house, and build a structure that you can say is a "house for the dead" for the child who did not stay. Place things in it that are from your family or that remind you of where you come from. Bring water and soil from your home, and provide things that will give the soul of your child a place to live so they do not need to live on inside your body or in your heart. Place the house somewhere no one else will ever see it, and leave it there.

Near where I live, a municipal cemetery has created a section called Little Spirits. It's a place to do a ceremony and create a house for an aborted, miscarried or stillborn child. Communities are starting to understand this tradition from long ago and are increasingly understanding the need to remember all children, even the unborn.

Twin Loss

Most women don't realize they are carrying twins or multiple babies. Why is this? It is thought that at least 85 percent of twins do not stay while the other twin lives on.[42] The departure of the second twin or other multiple children occurs very early in pregnancy, usually before eight weeks.[43] Children and adults don't always remember their twins or multiples — or if they do remember, they don't often talk about it — but they behave in ways that subtly indicate they are concerned for, and perhaps taking care of, another person, long after the unremarked death of their twin.

It is important to honour the twin who did not live as you would a single baby who miscarried. Families, including the twin who survives, will have feelings that need to be recognized, and they should be encouraged to express them. A ceremony, much like one for miscarriage, will help the family acknowledge the mystery and the many reasons why this child didn't live. This is also a powerful way to honour the child who does live. Often the children who live have a sense of death in and around them, and if they aren't told they had a twin, or if no one knew there was a twin, they may integrate the death as having something to do with them. They will mistake their sibling's death as a part of their own identity, and it will play out in their lives in a myriad of ways. Two valuable books on twin loss are Joan Woodward's *The Lone Twin: Understanding Twin Bereavement and Loss* and Althea Hayton's *Womb Twin Survivors: The Lost Twin in the Dream of the Womb*.

There are other circumstances where babies die: Abnormal chromosomes may be detected during pregnancy and the couple may decide to abort; babies may be born so prematurely that they cannot survive outside the womb, even with the help of the NICU; and some babies who are old enough to live, may not, even with the best of care. All these babies are real babies. Finding a way to honour them and honour parenthood are of utmost importance.

Summary

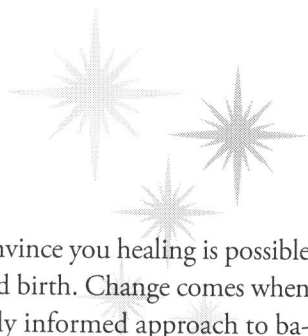

I hope you have now seen evidence that will convince you healing is possible despite the challenges surrounding pre-birth and birth. Change comes when we offer an emotionally attuned and historically informed approach to babies, and to adults who once were babies. By using the Family Field lens, we can gain an understanding of the past influences that have been inherited in the form of symptoms. And by re-examining the circumstances before conception, during pregnancy (particularly the first month), at birth, and just after birth, we can create a composite chart to connect our babies' or our own experience with the experiences of others in our ancestry.

Indicators of past trauma can be detected in all age groups. Once they are identified, they are highly responsive to tender words of regret that, if shared sincerely, will begin to unravel the protective coping strategies that developed in a baby or adult due to challenging early experiences. Babies, children, and adults will respond with grief, with anger, and even with joy that the past wound has finally been acknowledged. If verbal acknowledgement is not enough, osteopathy or craniosacral therapy may be warranted to further heal the emotional and physical impacts. Over time, often years, these painful early events will integrate, and life will feel easier. With sustained compassion and steady, persistent attention to their root causes, much change can come.

We've seen why it's important to do this work. Each stage of human development finds its foundation in earlier stages. Every one of our physiological systems will have formed by the end of the first month of pregnancy. How a mother and father feel about each other, this child, and their lives will shape how the baby's systems grow. Will the systems become efficient because they grow in an environment of ease? Or will they perform their functions with the memory of interruptions? If the prenatal or birth environment is full of added complexities, such as stress, poor diet, environmental toxins, or medical interventions, babies, children, and later adults will play out these complexities and interruptions in how they eat, sleep, learn, play, love, and complete tasks.

Because we grow into the patterns set for us by our early environment, we must return to that environment in order to find a new way today. This book provides an introduction to the work required for that return. Past and future intermingle in the therapeutic milieu. A forty-year-old man can experience his consciousness from three weeks after conception as though he is that age in the present. His body will feel small, he will feel surrounded by the feelings he had in the womb, and he will be open to finding a new way to live with that experience so it no longer unconsciously distracts and overwhelms him in the present.

Early stages of being an embryo, a fetus, a birthing baby, and newborn persist in us, and when we take a new step in our adult development that calls upon a foundation we missed at an earlier stage, we must go back, find the resources our earlier self missed, and give ourselves those needed resources. Then, as adults, we can progress with a more solid foundation underneath us. It's a magical thing.

We could say that pre-birth and birth are markers of society. What emphasis does a society place on family? And especially on the pregnant family? How loved and healthy babies and adults are reflects the resources that surround them. A mother who was a refugee at the time of her pregnancy will have that stress reflected in the birth of her child and in the way her child develops. The same stress will occur for a mother who may be resourced in some ways, but works in a high-pressure job. Her baby won't be able to tell the difference. Some children will have more innate resources than others, but nothing replaces communion, support, love, and access to clean water and healthy food.

If families and societies worldwide were to employ the perspectives held out in this book, we could see a global shift away from violence, addiction, and illness, particularly so-called mental illness. We could make it a priority for all families to receive craniosacral therapy or osteopathy in every hospital after birth, and in cases of birth interventions, for the first year and a half. Families could be educated about the short- and long-term consequences of pre-birth and birth interventions, supplying them with an advocate during birth so they can focus on birth itself.

Regardless of your approach after reading this book, I invite you to consider how the content applies to your own life and the lives of your loved ones. If nothing else, may you peer more deeply into your own and your fellow humans' present challenges. If you can imagine that others were also once babies, and might have been subjected to painful, threatening, or isolating experiences, you may find an extra measure of compassion or be able to offer perspective to their journey.

ACKNOWLEDGEMENTS

This book would be impossible without the families and individuals whose stories I'm privileged to tell. Many days of joyful life to them for their willingness to explore the unknown and emotionally charged terrain of pre-birth and birth content in a society that does not yet know how to thank them for their courage or show its remorse for their suffering.

My profound awe for the founders of pre-birth and birth inquiry, Carl Jung and Otto Rank, who, thanks to some unnamed wisdom and their own refreshing intelligence, picked up the quiet and inchoate call to continue the ancient, yet forgotten inquiry. And to those who dared to sustain public challenge and go further: Lietaert Pierbolte, Francis J. Mott, Nandor Fodor, R.D. Laing, Frank Lake, Elizabeth Fehr, Stanislav Grof, Lloyd De Mause, Joseph Chilton Pearce, and David Chamberlain, to name a few, whose bodies of work we learn eagerly from today. And then there are a dear few who have guided me in my personal explorations, either through therapy and/or illuminating conversation: William Emerson, Raymond Castellino, Wendy-Anne McCarty, Jaap van der Wal, Rupert Linder, Michael Trout, Myrna Martin, and Andrew Feldmar. A hearty bow to all practitioners in the Association of Prental and Perinatal Psychology and Health (APPPAH) and to my colleagues in the International Society for Pre- and Perinatal Psychology and Medicine (ISPPM). I would not know what questions to ask without your curiosity, findings, and organization.

I thank Audrey McClellan, a truly adept and kind editor, whose keen eye has smoothed and shaped these pages.

And finally, to my beloved Bruce, whose care for me midwifes all my creations.

NOTES

1. A more detailed exploration of how soul enters form goes beyond the scope of this book. The use of the term "soul" here is meant to acknowledge the level of ourselves that is unique from body and spirit.
2. Private Patient Files, 1999 – 2016, Vancouver, BC.
3. J. Upledger, *Somato Emotional Release* (Berkeley, CA: North Atlantic Books, 2002).
4. Cranial molding is a phenomenon in which the bones and membranes of the skull retain the shape of a traumatic event.
5. Private Patient Files 1999 – 2016, Vancouver, BC.
6. R. Linder, "Love, Pregnancy, Conflict, and Solution," *Journal of Prental and Perinatal Psychology and Health* 31, no. 2 (December 2016).
7. R. Castellino, *The Polarity Therapy Paradigm Regarding Pre-Conception, Prenatal and Birth Imprinting* (Santa Barbara, CA: Castellino, Prenatal and Birth Therapy Training, 1995); also M. Martin, "Module 1: Attachment," in the *Healing Early Developmental Trauma Video Series*, www.myrnamartin.net
8. Ibid.
9. Ibid.
10. Ibid.
11. Wal, J, van der, 2007. The Speech of the Embryo, *Biodynamic Craniosacral Therapy*, Vol. 1., pp. 83 – 102. North Atlantic Books, Berkeley, USA.

12. Wal, J, van der, 2007. "Human Conception: How to Overcome Reproduction?" in *Biodynamic Craniosacral Therapy,* Vol. 1. North Atlantic Books, CA., USA. pp. 137 – 54.

13. Wal, J, van der. "The Embryo in Us" — A Phenomenological Search for Soul and Consciousness in the Prenatal Body," *Journal of Prenatal and Perinatal Psychology and Health* 27, no. 3 (April 2013).

14. Private Patient Files, 1998 – 2008, Vancouver, BC.

15. Ibid.

16. Martin, "Module 1, Attachment."

17. Private Patient Files, 1998 – 2008, Vancouver, BC.

18. J. Boivin, L. Bunting, J.A. Collins, and K.G. Nygren, "International Estimates of Infertility Prevalence and Treatment-Seeking: Potential Need and Demand for Infertility Medical Care," *Human Reproduction* 22, no. 6 (2007): 1506 – 12, http://humrep.oxfordjournals.org/content/22/6/1506.short

19. At the time of the writing of this book, new developments in ART have extended the time a blastocyst can live outside the mother. By creating an environment that mimics the mother's endometrium in the lab, the blastocyst can survive up to fourteen days outside the mother's body.

20. Private Patient Files, 1998–2008, Vancouver, BC.

21. Ibid.

22. Castellino, *The Polarity Therapy Paradigm.*

23. Ibid.

24. Umbilical affect is a phenomenon affecting digestion and emotional and physical stability in a baby or child as a result of trauma at the umbilicus.

25. J. Piek, *Infant Motor Development* (Champaign, IL: Human Kinetics, 2006).

26. Private Patient Files, 1998 – 2008, Vancouver, BC.

27. Classical embryological texts will describe the "middle" as the "mesoderm." My choice to not use this term is thanks to embryologist Jaap van der Wal's philosophy and finding that the middle layer of an embryo is not an epithelium, as signalled by the use of the root "derm." Rather, the middle gives rise to a centrally embedded tissue later giving rise to visceral, connective, fluid, tissue in which soul is believed to reside.

28. Jaap van der Wal, "Human Conception: How to Overcome Reproduction — A Phenomenological Approach of Human Fertilization," *Energy and Character* 33 (September 2004); van der Wal, "Human Conception: How to Overcome Reproduction?" in *Biodynamic Craniosacral Therapy*, 137 – 154.

29. R. Sheldrake, *The New Science of Life: The Hypothesis of Formative Causation* (London: Icon Books, 2009).

30. Private Patient Files, 1998 – 2008, Vancouver, BC.

31. T.W. Sadler, *Langman's Medical Embryology*, 10th ed. (Baltimore: Lippincott Williams & Wilkins, 2006).

32. C. Panthuraamphorn, "Environmental Influences on Human Brain Growth and Development," *Journal of Prenatal and Perinatal Psychology and Health*, 12, no. 3 – 4 (Spring/Summer 1998).

33. J. Herman, *Trauma and Recovery: The Aftermath of Violence* (New York: Basic Books, 1997).

34. Ibid.

35. Robert Oliver, "The Ideal Cesarean Birth," *Journal of Prenatal and Perinatal Psychology and Health*, 14, 3 – 4 (Spring/Summer 2000): 331 – 45.

36. Ibid.

37. Ibid.

38. Michel Odent, *Primal Health* (London: Century Hutchison, 1986).

39. R. Castellino and M. Jackson, lecture to the World APPPAH Congress, Los Angeles, CA, 2007.

40. Odent, Primal Health.

41. Heidelise Als, originator of the Newborn Individualized Developmental Care and Assessment Program (NIDCAP), has designed systems for NICUs that enhance connections between parents and their premature or unwell babies while in the Neonatal Intensive Care Unit after birth. These NICUs include private rooms, dimmed lighting, the clustering of care to allow the family to get rest, and more.

42. C.E. Boklage, "The Frequency and Survivability of Natural Twin Conceptions," in *Multiple Pregnancy: Epidemiology, Gestation and Perinatal Outcome*, 1st ed., ed. Louis G. Keith, Emile Papiernik, Donald M. Keith, et al. (New York: Taylor & Francis Group, 1998), 41 – 42, 49.

43. Private Patient Files, Vancouver, 2009.

RESOURCES

Therapy
BEBA: Building and Enhancing Bonding and Attachment www.beba.org
Ray Castellino www.castellinotraining.com
Emerging Families www.emergingfamilies.com
Myrna Martin www.myrnamartin.net
Foundations VIE www.foundationvie.org
Biodynamic Osteopathy www.jamesjealous.com/physician-directory/
International Association of Healthcare Practitioners
    www.iahp.com/pages/search/index.php
Jon RG & Troya GN Turner www.Whole-Self.org
    & www.Cosmoanelixis.gr Whole-Self Online University
Kelduyn R. Garland Innerconnections@innerconnections.us
Olga Gouni www.Cosmoanelixis.gr Whole-Self Online University

Organizations
Association for Prenatal and Perinatal Psychology and Health (APPPAH)
    www.apppah.org
International Society for Pre- and Perinatal Psychology (ISPPM)
    www.isppm.de
World Organization of Prenatal Education Associations (OMAEP)
    www.omaep.com
Foundation VIE www.foundationvie.org
Birthing The Future www.birthingthefuture.org
Touch The Future www.ttfuture.org

Whole-Self Discovery & Development Institute International, Inc. www.Whole-Self.org; www.Cosmoanelixis.gr Whole-Self Online University

Trainings
Ray Castellino www.castellinotrainings.com
Myrna Martin www.myrnmartin.net
Emerson Seminars www.emersontrainings.com
Birth into Being www.birthintobeing.com
Karuna Institute www.karuna-institute.co.uk
Foundation VIE www.foundationvie.org
Michael Shea Teaching www.michaelsheateaching.com
Association for Prenatal and Perinatal Psychology and Health www.birthpsychology.com
Arbeitskreis Psychosomatik Vorderpfalz www.schroth-apv.com
Body-Mind Centering www.bodymindcentering.com
Jon RG & Troya GN Turner www.Whole-Self.org
Olga Gouni www.Cosmoanelixis.gr Whole-Self Online University

Research Database
www.primalhealthresearch.com
www.wombecology.com
www.apppah.org

INDEX

(f) after a page number indicates an illustration
(n) after a page number indicates a note

V

vacuum extraction and forceps
    about, 95
    effects of, 96–7, 119
    healing processes, 95, 97–8, 119
van der Waal, Dr. Jaap
    egg and sperm union, 42–4
    egg consciousness, 41–2
    embryo and psyche, 42
    implantation, 58
    middle dimension, 65, 132 (n 27)
violence (imprint), 31–2
visualization, v–vi

Z

zygote, 42, 44, 57

ABOUT MIA KALEF

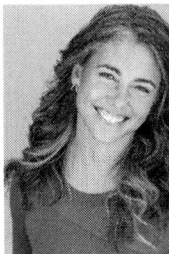

Mia Kalef is a therapist, author, and ceremonialist, dedicated to seeing the soul of things. She practiced as a Chiropractor for eighteen years and has been a craniosacral therapist for twenty-five years. She mentors health professionals in bringing prebirth and birth awareness into their work and gives divinations in the tradition of the Dagara people of west and central Africa. She lives on an island in the North Pacific with her husband Bruce, and works locally and internationally serving humanity's intersection with the subtle world. www.miakalef.com

29230763R00099

Printed in Great Britain
by Amazon